FERTILITY
WISDOM

FERTILITY WISDOM

HOW TRADITIONAL CHINESE MEDICINE CAN HELP OVERCOME INFERTILITY

ANGELA C. WU, LAc, OMD

with Katherine Anttila
and Betsy Brown

Notice

This book is intended as a reference volume only, not as a medical manual. The information given here is designed to help you make informed decisions about your health. It is not intended as a substitute for any treatment that may have been prescribed by your doctor. If you suspect that you have a medical problem, we urge you to seek competent medical help.

Mention of specific companies, organizations, or authorities in this book does not imply endorsement by the publisher, nor does mention of specific companies, organizations, or authorities imply that they endorse this book.

Internet addresses and telephone numbers given in this book were accurate at the time it went to press.

Book design by Joanna Williams

Library of Congress Cataloging-in-Publication Data

Wu, Angela C.
    Fertility wisdom : how traditional Chinese medicine can help overcome infertility / by Angela C. Wu, with Katherine Anttila and Betsy Brown.
        p.   cm.
    Includes index.
    ISBN 13 978–1–59486–137–6 paperback
    ISBN 10 1–59486–137–4 paperback
    1. Fertility, Human—Popular works.   2. Infertility—Alternative treatment—Popular works.
3. Medicine, Chinese.   I. Anttila, Katherine.   II. Brown, Betsy (Elizabeth Ann), date   III. Title.
RC889.W83   2006
616.6'9206—dc22   2006011574

Distributed to the trade by Holtzbrinck Publishers

2 4 6 8 10 9 7 5 3 1   paperback

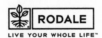

We inspire and enable people to improve their lives and the world around them

For more of our products visit **rodalestore.com** or call 800-848-4735

For my miracle babies, Devin and Robyn

CONTENTS

PREFACE

A WORD FROM A
WESTERN DOCTOR

It was 20 years ago when I first became intrigued by the science of fertility. A medical student at the time, I was fascinated by the role hormones play in human health, and with how they affect whether or not a woman conceives.

As my medical career progressed, I made fertility my specialty, and my choice has proven to be both timely and personally relevant. In the 15 years since I began my clinical practice—first in Seattle, now in San Francisco—I've seen infertility evolve into a high-profile medical issue confronted by more and more couples. According to the Centers for Disease Control and Prevention, in 2002, of the 62 million women of reproductive age in the United States, approximately 10 percent visited a doctor for advice or treatment related to infertility. And if the number of couples visiting my office is any indication—up to 500 new clients a year—the segment of the population seeking fertility support has only grown since then.

The source of this "epidemic," I believe, is largely cultural. It started with the Baby Boomer generation, with couples putting off childbearing by 10 to 15 years while they pursued careers. Today, many young women delay childbearing for various reasons. As their biological clocks tick, the quality of their eggs declines. In my practice, reduced ovarian reserve and "unexplained" infertility (often a function of egg quality) are the top two infertility diagnoses, followed by sperm disorders in men and endometriosis and Fallopian tube complications in women.

In addition to approaching infertility from a professional perspective, I've experienced firsthand the emotional and physical challenges couples face when they can't conceive the child they so desire. Without in vitro fertilization, my wife and I would not have our daughter. Our personal struggle with infertility makes me particularly sympathetic to what my clients go through when they come to me for advice and treatment.

Over the years, I have seen more clients take fertility into their own hands by exploring Traditional Chinese Medicine as a complement or alternative to Assisted Reproductive Technology (ART). Many of those women and their partners are also clients of Dr. Angela C. Wu.

At first I was skeptical about Traditional Chinese Medicine, but I took the time to visit with Dr. Wu to understand more about her work. I have to admit, I do not know why Traditional Chinese Medicine has a positive impact on infertility. I'm a physician trained in Western theories and protocols, and as you may discover as you read this book, it can be challenging to merge a Western medical mind-set with Eastern ways of perceiving human health.

What I do know is that there are things that Western science simply can't explain. I am open to the idea that "spirit"—though beyond the realm of Western medicine—plays a role in physical health. As Western medicine explores the importance of the mind-body connection in treating illness and keeping people vital, I think we will find that Traditional Chinese Medicine can contribute to our understanding of human health and fertility.

Victor Y. Fujimoto, MD
Reproductive Specialist
San Francisco

March 10, 2006

ACKNOWLEDGMENTS

I would like to acknowledge the contributions of a few people without whom this book would not exist.

- Rev. Ming-I Tsao, who took me into his home, taught me the complex art and science of pulse reading, and opened my eyes to the big picture of Taoism. I remember the day he read my pulses and told me I was destined to go overseas. At the time I found his prediction only amusing. Since then I have come to realize that, in teaching me to read pulses, he was preparing me for wisdom beyond the corporeal. An appreciator of good food (and an excellent cook), Rev. Tsao knew how to inspire and shape my mind by feeding my body.
- Dr. Shun Chiu, a general in the Chinese army, who taught me acupuncture. Watching him work was a revelation. A group of patients, complaining of headaches, would hold hands. Dr. Chiu would needle only the first person in line, and everyone would feel relief. A dedicated practitioner of meditation, Dr. Chiu was my inspiration in breaking with tradition; he would use only one needle, and leave it in for only a very short time. Today, honoring his wisdom in my clinic, I use fewer needles than many practitioners, and leave them in for less time.
- Dr. Yat-Chow Yeung, a well-known scholar in the Chinese community, who taught me the art and science of Chinese herbs. His pioneering wisdom transformed my perspective on healing by providing me with powerful new tools. Breaking with tradition, he honored me as his only female disciple—and the last disciple in a long life of teaching. He coached me through the challenges of working with HIV/AIDS patients in the 1980s. And when I would thank him for teaching me about Traditional Chinese Medicine, he would thank me for teaching him about people.

I remember when my beloved mentor—then in his 80s, his health failing—began to go blind and gave up his healing practice. One day, over a leisurely Chinese meal (our weekend tradition), I shocked him by saying: "You know, I'm a better doctor than you are . . ."—his face fell at the slight—". . . because I have had the privilege of better teachers." "You naughty girl!" he laughed. And, giving in to my insistence, he honored me again by accepting me as his doctor. Dr. Yeung took herbs according to my protocols and within a week, his vision improved and he felt strong enough to resume his own practice. I could tell he was happy, as I always could, because he patted me on the back—an affectionate departure from the strict "no touch" tradition between men and women in our culture at that time.

- Mantak Chia, whose dedicated efforts brought Taoist wisdom and practices to our modern world.

- Dr. George Araki, a true pioneer on the frontier where Western biological sciences meet Traditional Chinese Medicine and other alternative approaches to health and wellness. A Stanford-trained scientist who described himself as a "holistic biologist," Dr. Araki founded two groundbreaking interdisciplinary programs at San Francisco State University—the Center for Interdisciplinary Science and the Institute for Holistic Healing Studies. With his support, leadership, and friendship, I was able to found and direct SFSU's Chinese Healing Studies program—the first of its kind—bringing the concepts that underpin my fertility practice to a wider audience of future practitioners. Dr. Araki's amazing spirit and his huge heart live on in the work I do today, both healing and teaching.

- Nancy Merrell, who helped me overcome self-doubt and persuaded me that I *did* have a book in me.

- Clare Campbell, who patiently talked me through the concepts that became *Fertility Wisdom*.

- Stuart Kenter, who began the process of translating the fertility program I practice in my clinic into a book reaching out to a much broader audience.

- Kathy Anttila, for the great gifts of her time, talents, and support.

- Betsy Brown, whose words have given a clear, compelling, beautiful voice to the challenging concepts in this book, and whose steadfast friendship I treasure.

- Doug Abrams, who shepherded our writing team through the publishing process and whose own book so inspired me.
- Susan Berg, our gracious editor, whose patient and gentle touch has guided us on our journey, and whose sensitive vision for this book enabled us to create something in which we take great pride.
- The many clients who shared their stories, their lives, and their miracles with me—especially those whose experiences are documented in the pages that follow.
- My staff, without whose help there would be no miracle babies, and whose support, dedication, and hard work made writing this book possible.
- My friends and family. It's been said that friends are God's way of apologizing for the family given to us. In my life, there is no cause for apology: God has blessed me in both.

INTRODUCTION

THE MIRACLE WITHIN

If you've picked up this book because you are considering a pregnancy and want to maximize your chances of conceiving, congratulations! In your hands you hold tools to help you achieve what every expectant parent wants: a problem-free pregnancy and a healthy, happy new baby.

On the other hand, if you're reading because, despite your best efforts and deepest desires, the baby you hope to welcome hasn't arrived—have hope! You are not alone.

Maybe you're like Marcia*: For 13 years she tried unsuccessfully to conceive. Unable to find a medical reason for her lack of success, doctors gave Marcia a common and frustrating diagnosis: "unexplained infertility" . . .

Or Jane: High levels of follicle-stimulating hormone (FSH)—considered a sign of poor egg quality—gave her roughly a 5 percent chance of conceiving without a donor egg . . .

Or Tina: Entering menopause at age 50, with hot flashes, a fluctuating menstrual cycle, a deep desire to have a baby, and the clock ticking . . .

Or Naomi and Terry: With her right ovary removed and his sperm count low, they knew that, at ages 39 and 46 respectively, the odds of them conceiving a baby were low . . .

Or Louise: Suffering her first hot flash at age 25, diagnosed as premenopausal at 28, told at 30 that her hormone levels gave her zero chance of conceiving...

Or Lila: Her uterine lining was so thin that a fertility expert recommended she start looking for a surrogate mother if she wanted her own biological child . . .

Or Karen: After miscarrying at 42, she learned she had endometriosis

*Names that appear in *Fertility Wisdom* have been changed to protect privacy.

and uterine fibroids the size of Ping-Pong balls—a diagnosis that could cancel future hopes of pregnancy . . .

Or Jennifer: Ready to give up at 46, after seven miscarriages and five unsuccessful in vitro fertilization cycles.

Diagnosed as "infertile"—technically defined as the inability to conceive after 1 year of effort without contraceptives—these women and their partners represent what some have called an epidemic. With couples marrying later and trying to conceive later in life, infertility has become one of our most pressing health care concerns. In fact, today, one in five couples in the United States faces this daunting diagnosis.

But Marcia, Jane, Tina, Naomi and Terry, Louise, Lila, Karen, and Jennifer have more in common than discouraging medical diagnoses, failed pregnancies, and dim hopes of parenthood. They've beaten the odds, astonished their doctors, and realized their most cherished dreams by making their own miracles. They've conceived, carried, and delivered healthy babies, and they've done it by applying the practical wisdom you now hold in your hands, inspired by Traditional Chinese Medicine.

MIRACLES ON CLEMENT STREET

Although miracles like the ones just described can take place anywhere, our story begins in San Francisco, California, where I have maintained a practice in Traditional Chinese Medicine for nearly 30 years.

My clinic—Wu's Healing Center—is on Clement Street, in a bustling neighborhood of dim sum restaurants, Asian grocery stores, herb shops, and Chinese bakeries. Here we use a variety of Eastern tools and techniques—from acupuncture and herbs to acupressure and meditation—to help women (and men) strengthen, harmonize, and balance their bodies so that they can conceive and carry their babies to full term.

Step inside our clinic and you can't miss a wall-size collage dedicated to the babies doctors thought would never be born. We call the little miracles in this photo collage "acubabies": babies conceived and born, with support from acupuncture and other traditional Eastern therapies, often against tremendous odds. Their parents faced health challenges—from high FSH levels and polycystic ovaries to early menopause, to thin uterine lining, to sperm disorders, to unexplainable infertility—that placed them among the thousands of U.S. couples diagnosed as infertile every year.

In 2005 alone, our modest clinic helped 79 fertility-challenged women become pregnant—39 with support from Western reproductive technologies and 40 naturally. Twenty-nine of our female fertility clients were over the age of 40, and 14 of these women conceived naturally. Most of these women wondered if they would ever conceive at all.

HOPE—AND A HAPPIER PREGNANCY

Since our first American* acubaby was born in 1982, we've greatly refined our approach to infertility, adding new tools based in Traditional Chinese Medicine, adapting our approach to Western ways of thinking, often working in partnership with Western fertility experts, and creating a program that can be applied by hopeful parents like you—whether or not you work with a practitioner of Traditional Chinese Medicine.

The *Fertility Wisdom* we have developed—the same approach you will follow through the course of this book—has given our clients something they lacked when they came to our clinic: hope. It also delivers benefits well beyond an enhanced ability to conceive.

If women are using *Fertility Wisdom* in conjunction with Western technologies, such as in vitro fertilization, they find themselves better able to manage the physical discomforts and emotional stresses of these treatments. And when they do become pregnant, women who adhere to the concepts behind our *Fertility Wisdom* increase their chances of full-term pregnancy. They have more energy and vitality, less nausea, fewer mood swings, and a brighter outlook. When it comes time to deliver, labor often lasts 4 to 6 hours instead of days. Mothers bounce back without depression or fatigue

---

*I practiced Traditional Chinese Medicine in China before coming to the United States and was blessed with the opportunity to support pregnancies there, as well.

and with better long-term reproductive health. Babies are calmer, with more regular sleep patterns and fewer health concerns. And none of the babies born to mothers who have followed my recommendations—even older mothers—has been born with Down's syndrome.

Our *Fertility Wisdom* program has proven so successful that it has attracted the attention of an ever-growing number of clients and Western fertility experts. In fact, in 2001, I was invited to help with a study funded by the National Institutes of Health and conducted through the University of California—San Francisco's Fertility Experiences Project. The study followed 500 infertile couples for 18 months, assessing the psychological, financial, and social impacts of dealing with infertility. I provided the research staff with training on Traditional Chinese Medicine and my approach to enhancing fertility so that they could better understand and assess the experiences of couples taking an Eastern approach to infertility.

Even the media—local and national—has gotten involved, once dubbing me "the fertility goddess." I'm flattered, of course! But I'm also humbled, and a little bemused, because although her name is *not* Angela C. Wu, there *is* a fertility goddess behind the successful pregnancies our program nurtures.

INTRODUCING THE ORIGINAL CHINESE FERTILITY GODDESS

In our clinic we keep a small statue of a goddess named Quan Yin. Draped in flowing garments, beatific of countenance, toting a chubby child, and poised for miracles, Quan Yin is one of Buddhism's oldest and most beloved deities: the Goddess of Wisdom, Compassion, and Courage. She's also the patron saint of barren women, a virgin goddess with the power to grant children.

Quan Yin offers two additional gifts: She gives solace to the suffering, and she protects farmers and others whose lives are at the mercy of the elements—an apt extension of her expertise, when you consider that, from an

Eastern perspective, producing a baby is a lot like growing a garden.

Traditional Chinese Medicine views your body as a continuation of the natural world that surrounds it. Like the trees and flowers, fruits and vegetables that enrich our world, your body requires the appropriate environmental conditions in order to flourish. It needs gentle warmth, moisture, nourishment, and cultivation. And like a garden, your body is influenced by natural forces—wind, rain, snow, sunshine—conditions reflected both in your physical health and your emotional state.

As we work together through this book, our goal will be to help you establish an environment—physical, emotional, spiritual—that encourages conception. You'll learn to care for your body as you would a garden: preparing the soil, then planting the seed and nurturing it. You'll learn to establish and maintain good health defined by harmony, balance, and congruency. You'll discover how to balance Eastern fertility wisdom with Western Assisted Reproductive Technology (ART), if you choose. And you'll learn that by mirroring the qualities of Quan Yin—being compassionate and brave, wise and loving, attuned to the interplay of elements in the natural world—you can better prepare yourself to attract new life.

RISING PHOENIX: THE BLESSING OF REBIRTH AND RENEWAL

Every seed that sprouts in a field once deemed barren—every miracle baby—is the happy ending to one story and the exciting beginning of another. My son, my daughter, and the *Fertility Wisdom* program you are about to begin (itself a child of sorts) are no exceptions. Allow me to share the story of how all three seeds came to choose me as their garden.

I was born in China, into a culture that values women only for the heirs they give their husbands. Because they bring no honor to the family that bears them, daughters are tolerated rather than nurtured. (There's an old Chinese saying that sums it up: "You can snap a girl's neck, but she will still grow.") So when my father died not long after my birth, his family members, their grief unrelieved by a new baby girl, disowned my mother and me, and we returned to live with my mother's family.

As I grew, my mother and her stepmother, whom I called Ama, or grandmother, tried to show me my proper place, quiet and humble—a challenge, because I was an independent and inquisitive child. Ama, who practiced Traditional Chinese Medicine, constantly bombarded me with unsolicited health care advice: "Cover your head in winter!" "No cold drinks!" "Eat these special poached eggs after your period!" It would be many years before I recognized any kinship with Ama and her traditional medical wisdom.

In my grandfather, however, I found a kindred spirit with a soft spot for my adventurous nature. It was he who named me Rising Phoenix—the English translation of my Chinese name—he who taught me to love the countryside, and he who cultivated in me a variety of exhilarating but ungirlish interests, such as climbing trees.

Over time, I continued to find myself at odds with my culture's conception of a woman's place and potential. As a teenager, I decided that I would study the ancient art of Ba Zi, traditionally the domain of male scholars. Developed more than 5,000 years ago and based on the same concepts as the *I Ching,* Ba Zi assesses a person's potential path based on the position of the sun and moon in relation to the Earth at the time of one's birth. Ba Zi practitioners consult an esoteric and voluminous calendar called the *Wan Nian Li,* or *Ten Thousand Year Calendar,* to create a chart revealing the patterns—physical, emotional, spiritual—that will play out across one's lifetime.

Determined to learn from a renowned local Ba Zi master, I talked my way into a world few females inhabit by offering to keep house for the teacher while he conducted classes in his parlor. From the kitchen I would listen carefully as he revealed Ba Zi insights about how one's birth gives way to one's destiny. And on the way home, I would ride the bus with an older male student whose task it was to transcribe the day's lectures. When he complained of the work, I volunteered to take on the transcription for him, and I would work into the night to complete it (the teacher being none the wiser). In the process I absorbed Ba Zi like a thirsty young plant nourishes itself with water.

One day a Mongolian diplomat came to the teacher's house for a Ba Zi reading. As I served him tea, the diplomat jokingly asked what I saw in his past and predicted for his future. When, drawing on my secret Ba Zi knowledge, I offered particularly meaningful romantic insights and financial advice, the diplomat informed my teacher that he had a true Ba Zi scholar in his midst—disguised as a girl, perhaps, but a scholar all the same. To my great pleasure, I was allowed to join the study group with the men.

Eventually life led me away from such esoteric and unusual pursuits and back, at least temporarily, into the realm of tradition. Scandalized by my budding romance with an older musician (but that's another story), my mother's family arranged for me to marry a young man of their choosing. In my new husband's home, I was the traditional Chinese wife: obediently serving his favorite meals, putting his socks and shoes on him in the morning.

But outside the home, my independence could not be quelled. As a child, I'd held promise as a singer—I'd received training in Western-style opera—and as a young adult, I found work as the on-air hostess for a local radio station. When the radio station became a television station, there was plenty of opportunity for a bilingual young woman with a "good camera face," so I was sent to be trained for television. (To those who know me, it comes as no surprise that my specialties were soap opera ingénues—prone to romantic entanglements—and martial arts mavens.) At the same time, I developed an interest in Traditional Chinese Medicine and began to explore it.

One day, our soap opera was shooting a scene in Taiwan's famous Kending Park. Restless from the tedium of filming, I took advantage of a break to reveal a talent I'd been cultivating since childhood: I climbed a tree, just to show that I could. And as I made my leaping descent from the tree and rolled down a hill, I began to bleed. Without even realizing I was pregnant, I was having a miscarriage.

A few months later I was pregnant again, and I gave birth to a girl who lived only 42 days. A year later, my son Devin was born (4 agonizing weeks late), and my husband's family was overjoyed: I had produced not just an heir, but the first son of a first son—the fourth in the family.

One year and 1 week after Devin's birth, my daughter Robyn arrived. But after delivering Robyn, I continued to bleed. My blood pressure dropped precipitously, and I felt weak and adrift. Desperate, I made my husband promise that after my death he would take care of our children, especially our daughter, whom I feared leaving to a culture that would not value her as I did. I asked him to remarry, so my children would have a guiding female influence, but not to tell Devin and Robyn about their birth mother until they were grown.

I remember distinctly the sensations that followed. My mouth grew cold, and as that coldness spread, I felt my physical body dissolve. Suddenly I became aware of myself floating in the room. Below lay my body; above, a beautiful white light beckoned. I felt no sadness—just peace, joy, freedom—as I pursued the light, until I heard my own voice say, "I'm not ready yet." As sensation returned to my body, the noise of the hospital room filled my ears and I realized I was alive. But, although I had returned to a familiar body, my life would never be the same: Within a month of Robyn's birth, my husband informed me that he wanted a divorce in order to marry my best girlfriend, with whom he'd become involved.

Like many who have touched that white light for a fleeting moment, I resumed my life enriched by the perception that death is nothing to fear. But I also brought back a deep sense of mission, defined by my vulnerable new daughter, my fragile new independence, and the profound pain in my physical body. Though I had no idea where my mission would lead me, I committed myself to healing the female form to which I had returned—and to teaching my daughter to explore her full potential beyond the boundaries of traditional Chinese culture.

My recuperation was a long and difficult time during which I relearned every movement. Bedridden for weeks, I discovered that my hands naturally found their way to my poor abdomen, which had suffered so after Robyn's birth. As I meditated quietly in bed, I felt the warmth from my hands begin to heal my internal organs. Inspired by the healing power of my own Qi—the life force that inhabits each of us—I committed myself to applying the Traditional Chinese Medicine that had nurtured me (despite my protestations) as a child.

At first, much of my study was trial and error, using my own body as a laboratory. But as my knowledge, ambition, and strength increased, I continued my formal training. It proved an absorbing distraction after my divorce, and it empowered me to pursue my greatest passion: creating a better life for Devin and Robyn. (Although I could not be more proud of the adults they have become, I had begun to fear that Devin, coddled by his father's family, was becoming spoiled; and Robyn, ignored in favor of her brother, was withdrawing deeper and deeper into herself.) I completed my education in acupuncture and Traditional Chinese Medicine and established a practice through which I continued to question preconceived notions and test new approaches—including needling pregnant women, something traditional acupuncturists, steeped in centuries of tradition, simply didn't do. I moved to San Francisco, established a home, and earned permanent resident status in the United States. And finally, Devin and Robyn joined me.

Since coming to San Francisco, I have been blessed. In 1978, I opened my first Traditional Chinese Medicine clinic. In 1980, I founded the Chinese Healing Studies Program at San Francisco State University—the first program of its kind. And in the 1980s, when Western medicine was struggling to comprehend the AIDS epidemic, I dedicated myself to supporting people suffering from this devastating disease. Through it all, I was fortunate to work with countless clients, female and male, whose desire to conceive against all odds broadened my experience, expertise, and insight into the nature of infertility—and inspired me to make a specialty of fertility enhancement.

Together with these fertility clients, I've expanded the parameters of Traditional Chinese Medicine. (Many acupuncturists today will use needles to help women conceive, but still will not work on a woman while she is pregnant—a tradition I am working to help my colleagues transcend.) I've adapted ancient self-healing practices—meditation and acupressure—that for years were the exclusive domain of Taoist sages. I've interpreted Eastern concepts and tools to complement Western healing approaches and Western lifestyles and shared my perspective with Western fertility experts, like Dr. Victor Fujimoto, who authored the preface of this book. And I've formed healing partnerships with people who never cease to move me. Together we have proven that by challenging preconceived notions, we can reap unexpected benefits—among them, miracle babies—and pave the way for others on their own fertility journeys.

What began with my first American acubaby in 1982 has truly blossomed and born fruit, again and again, for me and for the families I am

TAKE YOUR FIRST STEPS

Throughout this book, you'll find exercises and meditation tips to help you culti-vate a positive attitude and a balanced emotional state conducive to conception and a healthy pregnancy. Ready to get started? Before you embark on our *Fertility Wisdom* program, sit in a quiet place without distractions, refresh yourself with a few deep breaths, and take the following first steps:

1. **Thank yourself.** Recognize the effort it took to pick up this book. Simply perusing these pages requires you to open your mind to new concepts and a new approach to your health. Acknowledge that effort as the sig-nificant first step toward success.

2. **Thank your body.** This trusty vehicle, chosen by your spirit before birth for your personal journey through life, has already carried you many miles. Close your eyes and bring your attention to your heart, your body's center of gratitude. Imagine a feeling of warmth and joy that begins in your heart and, with each beat of your pulse, permeates your body. Now smile—it's a simple but powerful act that, science has shown, can actually make you feel better! This joy, this attitude of gratitude and respect, is something we will cultivate throughout this program. You can start now.

3. **Paint a positive picture.** Here's a simple exercise that taps the power of positive thinking and visualization: Close your eyes and breathe comfort-ably. Smile! Then imagine the rewards you seek. What will your picture of success look like? Are you healthy and pregnant? Snuggling a happy baby? As you hold this image in your mind's eye, notice every element of it. What colors or objects—note their size and shape—do you see? What is the expression on your face? What emotions do you feel?

    Take a moment to treasure this image. Then exhale once more and open your eyes. If, at any time during your efforts to conceive, you find yourself losing confidence in a positive outcome, conjure up this picture of success—the colors, the sensations, the images. Experiencing what you want, if only in your imagination, is the first step toward making it real.

4. **Abandon preconceptions.** In my work with couples struggling to conceive, I have found that the most challenging people to help are those whose preconceptions leave little room for new ideas. Before you continue with this book, please, "empty your cup" of what you think you know so that I may fill it with a new and invigorating blend of pregnancy tea. Perhaps on first taste you'll find my brew too bitter or too sweet. But if you never empty your cup so that I may serve you, you'll never find out.

blessed to have watched take shape. May the pages that follow likewise enrich your life.

APPRECIATING THE GIFT

In the Taoist spiritual tradition into which I was born, life is a gift. It is up to us to learn to receive it, and when we do, we must treat it with gratitude.

I believe these guidelines apply to the life you lead and to the new life you wish to attract. You see, in Taoist tradition, our mothers and fathers don't choose us; we choose them. It is not for us, as hopeful parents, to decide which young spirit we will nurture, or when it will arrive. We can, however, make our bodies a welcoming place for new life to grow—balanced, harmonious, fertile.

So, whether you're reading this book as a first step toward pregnancy or to overcome seemingly insurmountable odds—roll up your sleeves and get ready to garden! With these tools, an open heart, and a little help from Quan Yin, you can do more than leave your fertility to chance. *You can make your own miracle.*

 WELCOME, GENTLEMEN!

Although in my practice, I have found that women most often take the initiative to seek support with infertility, it is not just a women's issue. (In fact, statistics show that as many as 15 percent of men between the ages of 15 and 50 struggle with infertility; some estimates say that roughly 30 percent are "subfertile.") Therefore, while chances are high that you, reader, are female, I wish to make it perfectly clear that my invitation to explore *Fertility Wisdom* extends to men as well. As you will learn as you continue reading, many of the exercises and recommendations in our program can and should be used by women and men alike to improve their general health and chances of conceiving. So although I generally will address myself to female readers (directing the occasional comment to men), ladies—please share the wisdom. Gentlemen are welcome. (After all, without their participation in some form, there will be no babies!)

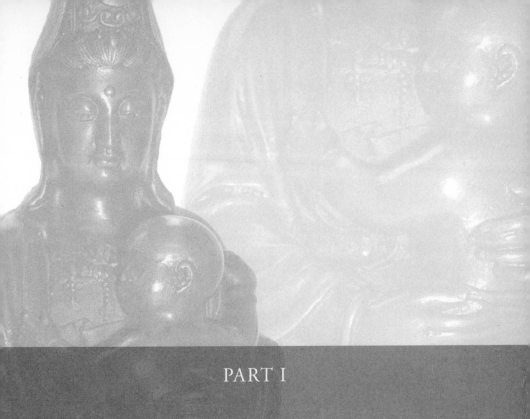

PART I

BEGINNING
THE
JOURNEY

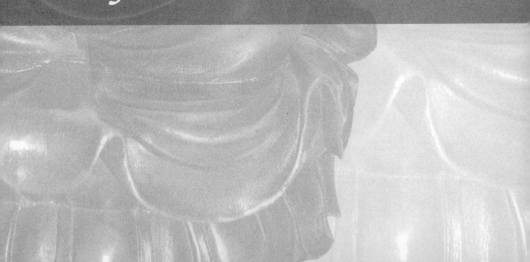

Adopting a new approach to the challenge of conceiving and carrying a baby against the odds takes an open mind, a willing heart, and the courage to follow a new path.

In Part I of your journey toward *Fertility Wisdom,* you will embark in a new and possibly unfamiliar direction, first exploring the Taoist philosophy that informs every recommendation and exercise in this book, then looking at its application in Traditional Chinese Medicine. You'll learn a quick and easy way to monitor your body's "weather" as it changes with the seasons and the impact of daily activities. Then, by completing a questionnaire similar to one I use in my clinic, you (and your partner) will assess your health, your attitude, and the factors that support or hinder your efforts to conceive.

Later in this book, we will take a step-by-step approach to preparing your body to welcome a baby. As your journey continues, get ready to:

- Take a whole new approach to eating and drinking—preparing the garden inside of you for pregnancy by avoiding food and drink with a negative impact on your ability to conceive. (Be willing to open your mind—these guidelines are very different from the Western nutritional principles you've followed your whole life!)
- Use acupressure to clear your internal organs of energy blockages that occur through negative emotions, stress, or overwork—and that can keep you from conceiving.
- Meditate, using images and sounds, to improve the flow of energy through your body and cultivate a frame of mind conducive to pregnancy.
- Strengthen your mind as well as your body's outer structure through exercises similar to Tai Chi, to help you prepare for conception and pregnancy.
- Learn how an herb called moxa can help you enhance your fertility by circulating your body's vital energy to key locations.
- Create home and work environments that support conception.
- Work with a practitioner of Traditional Chinese Medicine. Though

this is not necessary to follow our *Fertility Wisdom,* it's highly recommended to enhance the benefits of our program and tailor it to your personal constitution.

* Partner with your Western doctor or fertility specialist.
* Enhance the results and reduce the side effects of Western fertility treatments.

Now, please empty your cup.

 EMPTY YOUR CUP

The student traveled far to consult with the wisest of teachers, keeper of the secrets of life. Atop the highest mountain, in a humble shack, the student found the sage. "Tell me the purpose of your visit," said the sage, pouring the student a cup of tea.

"I have apprenticed myself to the world's best instructors, read volumes, memorized every lesson, and tested my skills against the brightest minds," the student replied. "I know the laws of nature, man, and the universe. What can I learn from you—an old hermit?"

As the student spoke, the old sage poured . . . and poured . . . and poured . . . until the tea overflowed onto the table, then the floor.

"Stop!" cried the student. "Can't you see that the tea is overflowing?"

"Yes, I see," said the sage, "that I cannot serve you, because your cup is already full."

CHAPTER 1

HARMONIZING
WITH NATURE

Before we go any further together, do one thing: Go outside. Find a place where you can anchor your feet on real soil, ideally in a garden. Plant yourself solidly and breathe in deeply, from the soles of your feet all the way up through your legs and body to the top of your head, nourishing yourself with the environment that surrounds you.

Now take a minute to glance around. Notice where there is sunlight and where there is shade. Imagine how these patterns of light and shadow might change throughout the day as the sun shifts in the sky. Now bring your attention to the weather: Does it feel warm or cool? Dry or damp? Is the air still? Is there a slight breeze? Or is it windy?

Continuing to breathe deeply from your feet, close your eyes and notice any sensations in your hands. Now bring your attention to your thoughts and emotions. What preoccupations have you brought to the garden? Are you still mulling over personal or work issues? What is your mood? Are you happy, sad, angry, worried?

Now bring your attention to the crown of your head. Imagine your personal energy reaching up to connect with the energy of the cosmos. Bring this cosmic energy in. Feel the connection between the Earth under your feet, your body, and the universe above you. Then, over the course of a few more breaths, let go of all emotions, all worldly concerns, all sensations—simply release them with each exhalation—until your mind and body are calm and empty. Before you open your eyes and return indoors, bring your hands to your navel. Be aware of the space you've just cleared and, in it, plant a tiny seed of hope—a prayer for what you would like to achieve.

Through your body, you have just experienced all the wisdom you need to move forward with this book. Now, so your mind can embrace what your body already understands, we will talk a little about Taoism, the philosophy that gave birth to Traditional Chinese Medicine, and the concepts of nothingness, balance, congruency, and harmony. Cultivating these states in your mind and body is vital to creating an environment that will attract new life.

Should you take the time to understand the thinking behind this new approach to fertility? Yes—because Western minds, accustomed to cause-and-effect analysis, often want to know "why." Understanding the Eastern perspective, even just a little, will make it easier to embrace the advice in the pages ahead and apply it effectively.

TAOISM: CREATING SOMETHING FROM NOTHING

Taoism is a system of beliefs, born over the centuries from Chinese philosophers' observations of the natural world, that informs every aspect of Chinese culture.* Religion, philosophy, art, literature, theater, ethics, politics, medicine—all grow from "the Tao," which, literally translated, means the path, or the way.

As followed in everyday life, the Tao leads us to health, happiness, and harmony with the cosmos. People who practice Taoism tap into the wisdom

---

*I'd like to point out here that the sexist limitations I experienced as a girl born in China, where female children are not valued as males are, grow from traditional Chinese culture but not from Taoist philosophy. As a Taoist, I believe men and women are very different in many ways—body, emotions, and talents. (That's why our *Fertility Wisdom* program includes slightly different guidelines for men and women.) But our strengths complement each other. By valuing the opposite sex's strengths and working together, I believe, we can create a society in which female and male energies (as you will learn, Yin and Yang) are balanced—an ideal worth working toward.

REMEMBER THE GARDEN

As you move forward with this book, please remind yourself that your body is like the garden in which you have just experienced the continuum of being. As in all gardens, the seed we hope to plant in our bodies grows best when we cultivate the ground and plant and nurture the seed in harmony with the laws of nature. You wouldn't put a tender plant in clay soil without first tilling and amending the earth—at least not if you wanted to give that plant its best start. You wouldn't plant in the dead of winter, or in the dry season without water, or in a sunless place. Likewise, if we tend our bodies, minds, and spirits with an awareness of the laws of nature, we improve our chances of welcoming the gifts of Quan Yin, the fertility goddess.

of the Tao by consulting the *I Ching,* or *Book of Changes,* an ancient oracle and one of the primary documents of Taoist thought. But we can also connect with the Tao through our bodies, by using the eating and drinking guidelines, meditation techniques, and exercises recommended later in this book.

Like many philosophies, Taoism holds at its core a belief about how the universe was formed. In Taoist thought, the material universe as we know it grew from a dynamic void called *Wu Chi.* Some people think of Wu Chi as God or Eternity—a power or a place beyond the plane of human existence. But a more meaningful interpretation of Wu Chi is "nothingness"— a sort of energized emptiness that holds the potential for creation.

Wu Chi, or nothingness, is more than just an interesting concept at the core of Traditional Chinese Medicine. It's a model for us to follow as we prepare your body for pregnancy. Remember the story about the sage, the student, and the overflowing cup, and the exercise in which you "emptied your cup" in order to partake of a new approach to fertility? Both this parable and practice are expressions of Wu Chi. They ask you to cultivate in yourself the dynamic void that is the source of all new life. By clearing out preconceptions and connecting with the primordial emptiness that gave birth to the universe, we create a space in which *something* may flourish.

Here's another way to look at it: When you cut open an apple, you find a seed. It doesn't look like an apple. It doesn't taste like an apple. It is not an apple. It is the potential—the nothingness—from which an apple tree grows. It is a prayer for apples.

YIN AND YANG: BALANCING OPPOSITES

The dynamic emptiness of Wu Chi gave birth to *Tai Chi,* the fundamental energy of the material world. Tai Chi is the union of two complementary opposites, *Yin* and *Yang.* Bringing these two elements into balance in our bodies is key to establishing an environment that welcomes new life.

In the Chinese language, the terms Yin and Yang originally referred to the shady and sunny sides of a mountain. Together they make up the entire mountain. Each side has the capacity for darkness and light as the sun moves in the sky—a phenomenon you experienced when, at the beginning of this chapter, you envisioned how the shifting sun might affect patterns of shade and light in the garden over time.

If you were to observe the garden across a long period of time, you would witness the continual transformation of day into night into day, with light giving way to darkness and darkness yielding to the light of a new day. This

---

 THE FIVE PRINCIPLES OF YIN AND YANG

In Chinese thought and medicine, there are Five Principles that govern the nature and interaction of Yin and Yang:

- All things have two aspects: Yin and Yang.
- Yin and Yang can be further divided into Yin and Yang. (Yin itself is composed of Yin and Yang elements, as is Yang.)
- Yin and Yang create each other.
- Yin and Yang control each other.
- Yin and Yang become each other.

FROM WU CHI TO TAI CHI—THE EVOLUTION OF YIN AND YANG

According to the Tao, the nothingness of Wu Chi makes room for Tai Chi, which is made up of Yin and Yang. In the familiar Tai Chi symbol—a circle that is half dark and half light—the Yin component (dark) contains the seed of Yang (light), just as Yang contains the seed of Yin.

From a Taoist perspective, the same natural forces that created the universe and shape the natural world around us come into play every time a baby is conceived and grows. The dynamic emptiness of Wu Chi is like the human womb, ready for Yin and Yang (egg and sperm) to unite to create new life. As the tiny embryo develops, the organ known as the Triple Warmer is formed, representing the Three Treasures. Five organ systems take shape, representing the Five Elements. And 12 acupuncture meridians (energy pathways), with a total of 365 acupuncture points, come into being, representing the 12 months and 365 days of the year.

process of perpetual, natural change is the very essence of Yin and Yang. Darkness, or Yin, always contains an element of light waiting to emerge. And light, or Yang, embodies the potential for darkness.

As twin pillars of Traditional Chinese Medicine, Yin and Yang have distinct qualities that manifest in the human body and psyche, as well as in the world around us. Yin, the shady side of the mountain, is associated with cold, rest, darkness, receptiveness, decrease, quiet. In the female/male equation that creates new life, Yin is the female component, the mother. It is completion and fruition. Yang, the sunny side of the mountain, is associated with heat, brightness, stimulation, activity, excitement, vigor, increase, arousal, beginning. It is the male counterpart, the father, to Mother Yin.

Your goal, through our work together, is to create an environment that is neither Yin nor Yang—neither too cool and damp nor too warm and dry—but a healthy balance of the two. The first step is to acknowledge that your body is not a finite, immutable system, but one in which change is constant. As you will learn, we can influence that change and increase our chances of conceiving through the foods we eat and the fluids we drink, as well as through meditation and exercise.

THREE TREASURES: CREATING CONGRUENCY AMONG HEAVEN, EARTH, AND HUMAN

In Chinese culture, we believe that the cosmos consists of three levels of being.

- **Heaven:** realm of the planets, of universal wisdom and energy, and of spiritual power
- **Earth:** the material world that grounds and nourishes us, the source of our most primitive knowledge and generative power
- **Human:** the in-between level, with access to both Heaven above and Earth below, the source of human power

Humans are endowed with the tools to tap each of these levels of being. Through our minds—instruments of intellectual thought, analysis, and moral action—we gain access to the treasures of Heaven: the universal wisdom of the cosmos and the satisfaction of a spiritual connection with all things. Through our hearts—the center of emotion in Eastern as well as Western cosmology—we can experience the treasures of the Human realm, including happy human relationships. And through the organs in our gut—liver, kidneys, stomach, bowels, reproductive organs—we can connect with the treasures of Earth: our primordial instincts, our ancestors.

The challenge we face every day of our existence is to live a life in which Heaven, Earth, and Human levels are aligned, or *congruent*. That means that the intent we generate in our minds is in synch with the intent of our hearts and the action of our guts.

Here's an example of congruency: In our minds, connecting us to Heaven, we know we want a baby in our lives, and we are committed to using our powers of reason, ingenuity, and understanding to achieve our goal. In our hearts, our link to Human gifts, we are open to loving a child, and to doing the hard work that every positive relationship (particularly one that lasts a lifetime) requires. And in our guts, our often-overlooked body-brain and our connection to the Earth, we are committed to securing the practical resources that will free us of stress, negative emotions, and primitive fears—often the source of imbalance, disharmony, and illness that can prevent us from conceiving.

The Heaven-Earth-Human paradigm has even more direct relevance to the issue of fertility and conception. In a graceful dance that mimics the very formation of the universe from Wu Chi, in the dynamic void that is the human womb, Heaven (sperm) and Earth (egg) align to manifest on the Human level as a baby.

THE FIVE ELEMENTS: HARMONIZING WITH NATURE

Look at the world around you, and, like the ancient Chinese sages who conceived of Taoism, you will see that life on Earth is composed of *Five Elements:* Wood, Fire, Earth, Metal, and Water.

Taoists believe that these Five Elements are the building blocks of all life, manifesting in our bodies as they do in our environment. In fact, every living thing is defined by its unique combination of Wood, Fire, Earth, Metal, and Water. The particular combination of these elements within each of us—established, Taoists believe, at the time of our birth—determines how we respond physically and emotionally to all of the forces of nature. It defines our health, and our fertility.

For good health and good fortune, we need both Yin and Yang versions of each of the Five Elements in our lives. When one or more elements dominate or are absent, health and fertility can be compromised; when all Five Elements are in harmony, our chances of conceiving improve. Note that we can determine our own distinct elemental patterns and the energies accessible to us by virtue of our birth date through the practice of Ba Zi, with its *Ten Thousand Year Calendar.* Based on the position of the stars, Ba Zi uses an ancient form of numerology to identify the relationship of the elements at the moment of our birth—for example, which elements we have more of, and which we have less of or lack altogether. (To learn more about Ba Zi, see the reading list in Appendix A on page 201.)

GETTING TO KNOW YOUR GUT BRAIN

Have you ever noticed that your body seems to know you're stressed before your mind grasps the source of your troubles? From the Taoist perspective, we owe this body-based awareness to our "gut brain," which connects us to the Earth level of the *Three Treasures (Heaven, Human, Earth).*

Lest you think it's only a figment of the Taoist imagination, please note that Western medicine also acknowledges the existence of your gut brain. Deep within your esophagus, stomach, small intestine, and colon lies your enteric nervous system—a complex physiological network that connects, through your central nervous system, to the brain in your head. A distant relative of the primitive "reptile brain" that guides less-evolved creatures, the gut brain reacts when we experience stresses that provoke our "fight or flight" response—and in modern life, that could be anything from a traffic jam to an argument with a loved one. When we're worried, stressed, angry, fearful, or depressed, our gut brain knows and tells us in the only way it can—through our gut.

What happens when you consistently ignore the messages of your gut brain? Maybe you forget to eat breakfast, ignoring the grumbling from below. Maybe you ignore the fact that raw broccoli gives you gas, or that you feel strangely chilled after eating ice cream—failing to make a connection between what you feed your body and the way it makes you feel. Maybe you ignore stresses at work, telling yourself to be tough or patient without acknowledging how you really feel. Over time, such behavior can harm your organs and result in chronic disharmonious health. Perhaps you experience constant constipation, diarrhea, or an ever-changing combination of the two—conditions that tell us that, perhaps, you must tend to your lifestyle as well as your body before you're ready for your baby.

The next time you feel constipated or cramped with diarrhea, listen to your gut brain. Was it really just "something you ate," or is this helpful organ sending you a message about the way you're living your life or treating your body? Trace the problem to its source. Use your heart (your Human brain) to identify the emotion you're experiencing. Use your head (your Heaven brain) to figure out a reasonable solution. And use your gut (your Earth brain) to guide you in practical action. Follow this approach, engaging all Three Treasures, whenever you face a challenge—whether it's honestly assessing how much you can get done during a day or dealing with a daunting diagnosis of infertility. How does this challenge make you feel? And what, practically, can you do about it?

As you'll see from the chart in Appendix B on page 205, each of the Five Elements is associated with a season of the year, organs in our bodies, a particular color and flavor, and time of day, demonstrating Taoism's belief in the interrelatedness of all things. These associations will be useful as—using food and drink, exercise, meditation, and other tools—we balance the Five Elements in your body for optimum fertility.

The Five Elements that, in combination, determine our personality, our constitution, our fertility, and our destiny are:

Wood. Present in the plants and trees that emerge, green, from dormancy in Spring, Wood represents the beginning of new life. The liver, which turns food into fuel that feeds the body's muscles, tendons, and ligaments, is one organ of the Wood element. One way we can assess the health of the liver is to look at the eyes, the exterior organ associated with Wood. Wood, which governs the body's nervous system, represents the creative urge to achieve and the ability to plan and make decisions. If you have difficulty initiating creative projects or tend to be indecisive, it may be that Wood is out of harmony in your body.

Fire. Whenever you feel the heat of the sun in Summer, enjoy the warmth of human relationships, admire the stars at night, or feel enthusiasm that inspires you to action, you're experiencing the Fire element. The ultimate in Yang energy, Fire symbolizes combustion and represents the natural world and our body functions at their peak. The heart is one of the organs associated with Fire; to assess its health, we look at the tongue. Fire also governs the circulatory system. If you have trouble feeling or expressing love or taking direct action in your life, Fire may be out of harmony in your body.

Earth. Abundance, harvest, nourishment, fertility—the bounty of Late Summer—represent the Earth element. Earth is considered critical to our ability to maintain balance. It symbolizes stability and consolidation and is associated with the spleen and the digestive system; we assess its health by looking at the mouth. If you experience constant digestive problems or are troubled by feelings of panic or worry, Earth may be out of harmony in your body.

Metal. To understand the Metal element, think of the minerals within the Earth, the force of gravity, and the powers of electricity and magnetism. By applying other elements, we can shape Metal into useful tools—for example, transforming iron into steel and steel into everything from an ax blade to a fine-edged scalpel through the power of Fire. Metal, at its peak in the Fall, represents cutting, editing, reshaping. It is associated with the lungs and the respiratory system, the nose, the skin, and the immune system. When Metal is out of harmony, you may experience frequent colds, allergies, or skin problems, or sadness or depression.

Water. The source of all life on Planet Earth, Water makes up much of the body and is critical to the health of our cells. The element of Winter, Water is represented by our vital fluids: blood, lymph, mucus, semen. It is flexible and powerful—able to flow into gaps or wreak destruction through floods. The ultimate in Yin energy, it represents potential. It is associated with the kidneys, bladder, and ears and governs the urinary and reproductive systems. When Water is out of harmony, you may have urinary tract or reproductive problems or be plagued by insecurity, fear, or timidity.

THINK POSITIVE

You've heard about the power of positive thinking. Here's a simple way to put it into practice by affirming your potential for fertility. Instead of focusing on any obstacles you perceive between you and pregnancy, imagine yourself prepared to conceive, even as you're taking steps to realize that dream. Find three times during your day—morning, midday, and evening—to remind yourself that you have, within you, the potential to achieve your goal. Repeat the following affirmations while visualizing symbols of the Tao's support.

SAY . . .	SEE . . .
I am open.	Wu Chi symbol (an empty circle)
I am whole.	Tai Chi symbol (Yin and Yang in balance)
I am congruent.	Pick three images that symbolize Heaven, Human, and Earth to you. Imagine them in perfect alignment.
I am harmonious.	Visualize the Five Elements—Wood, Fire, Earth, Metal, and Water—collaborating to create the perfect weather.

Relationships among the Five Elements

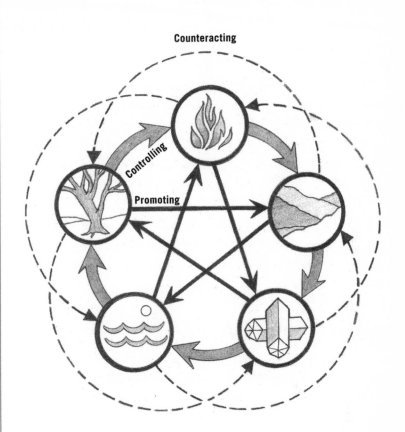

In our bodies and in the world around us, the Five Elements are interconnected in a perpetual cycle through which they give energy to and receive energy from each other.

Sometimes the relationships between elements are supportive, or promoting: For example, the presence of Water enhances Wood, just as gentle rain helps plants grow. Sometimes these relationships are restrictive, or controlling: For example, Metal tools, such as pruning sheers, can be used to shape and control the growth of a tree, a representative of the Wood element. At other times, elements may counteract each other: For example, although Metal can be used to shape Wood, an excess of Wood may overcome Metal's controlling influence—if you try to cut down a large tree with a pocket knife, you will end up with a very dull pocket knife.

This illustration shows the promoting, controlling, and counteracting relationships that exist among the Five Elements. Can you see how these relationships provide opportunities for us to restore harmony to our bodies—for example, controlling disharmonious Water (dampness) by adding warmth (Fire)?

NEXT STEPS: PUTTING THEORY INTO PRACTICE

Now that you've explored the often-puzzling wisdom of the Tao and begun to assess its impact on your life, where do we go from here? In the chapters ahead, we will apply these principles to your health and your lifestyle. We will take steps to restore the balance between Yin and Yang in your body. We will consider whether you are truly tapping the powers of the Three Treasures or are not congruent in your intentions, feelings, and actions—or are out of synch with your partner. We will take steps to create life-giving internal weather that reflects harmony among the Five Elements. And by replacing preconceptions with hope and prayer, replacing fullness with openness, we will conjure Wu Chi to make more room for a baby.

Katy and Brogan's Story
MIRACLE GIRLS

*I*t was 1976, and Tom was in graduate school when he and Susan married. They thought it best to wait a year, when they would be more settled, to have a child together. Besides, they had Luke, Susan's 6-year-old from a previous marriage—and all the time in the world to expand their family. Little did they know the challenges they would face when they made conception their goal.

Tom and Susan had been trying for a year and a half when they sought help from a Western fertility specialist. Tests revealed no problems with Tom's sperm. So Susan tried hormone treatments and a variety of insemination methods. Still she couldn't get pregnant. It wasn't until the couple had invested 3 years in Western fertility treatments that doctors realized the extent of their problem: After Luke's birth, Susan's cervix hadn't healed. Doctors had cauterized the cervix to speed things along—and in the process, destroyed the glands that produce the cervical mucus necessary for conception. Susan vividly remembers how her fertility specialist responded after discovering the cause of Susan's infertility: He handed her the business card for an adoption agency.

Living in student housing at the time, Susan shared her woes with a neighbor who was having trouble with her own pregnancy. At the neighbor's suggestion, the two women decided to seek help from Traditional Chinese Medicine, and they came to see me.

I still remember those early meetings with Susan. Loaded with hormones from her Western fertility treatments, she felt unbalanced. Her menstrual cycles were erratic, with spotting between periods. As she poured out her saga, I could hear frustration and fear—but I also heard intense commitment to doing whatever was necessary to bring a baby into her life. A check of Susan's vital signs from an Eastern perspective revealed a challenged constitution, but not one beyond hope. When I told Susan I thought we could indeed increase her chances of conceiving by bringing her body into balance and harmony, she said it was the first good news she'd heard in 5 years.

As Susan and I worked together and she embraced our Fertility Wisdom—from eating and drinking guidelines to meditation, acupressure, and exercise—the spotting stopped and she started to have regular periods. She began to feel her energy return. I remember the day I told Susan that her body presented a compelling invitation to conception. Now it was up to her baby to choose her. Two weeks later Susan was pregnant naturally and, in due time, Katy—the first child in the United States conceived with support from my fertility enhancement program—was born.

A few years later, after her son Luke died in a tragic accident, Susan returned to the clinic for help with her grief. In our conversations, she revealed that she and Tom had been trying for another child before Luke died. Could I help her conceive again? As she evolved through the phases of her grief, we gradually shifted our emphasis to improving her fertility, much as we had done before. With help from Traditional Chinese Medicine and high-tech

Western techniques, Brogan was conceived and born. Both girls are tickled to know that they were miracles of Traditional Chinese Medicine: my first American acubabies. To their mother—who, 25 years later, still has that adoption agency card—they remain nothing less than miraculous.

CHAPTER 2

OVERCOMING DISHARMONY

Now that we've explored the philosophical foundations of Eastern medicine, let's look more closely at how Traditional Chinese Medicine regards the phenomenon of infertility. We'll start by exploring some of the most common Western diagnoses I see in my San Francisco clinic. We will talk a little about Eastern methods of assessing and naming illnesses. Then, for a moment, we'll put aside whatever Western diagnosis you may have received—high FSH? low sperm count or motility? early menopause? unexplained infertility? thin uterine lining or poor egg quality?—and look at your body the way a practitioner of Traditional Chinese Medicine might, as a microcosm of the natural world, with its own weather.

WEST AND EAST: TWO PERSPECTIVES, TWO PATHS TO HEALTH

Western medicine and Traditional Chinese Medicine follow different paths to the same destination: good health.

In general, a Western physician diagnoses illness based on the patient's complaints and treats it by applying solutions that have worked on other patients with the same symptoms. A practitioner of Traditional Chinese Medicine also listens to the patient's complaints, but before she prescribes a course of treatment, she also checks the patient's weather.

31

YOUR BODY'S WEATHER REPORT: INVESTIGATING AND ASSESSING

Remember the exercise you completed at the beginning of Chapter 1 when, standing in the garden, you used your senses to assess the weather? Was the garden warm or cool, dry or damp? Was the air fresh or stagnant, windy or still?

These are the same questions a practitioner of Traditional Chinese Medicine would ask about your body when diagnosing your condition. She would explore your health—top to bottom, inside and out—using five traditional methods of investigation:

- **Asking:** A practitioner of Traditional Chinese Medicine will inquire about your life and your health.
- **Observing:** She will note both your appearance—including face, eyes, and tongue—and behavior.
- **Smelling:** Does your breath or your body have a fresh or stagnant odor? Sweet or acrid? (Each odor gives different clues about your personal weather pattern—especially when you're under stress.)
- **Listening:** Your practitioner will listen not only to what you say, but also to the exact words you choose; to the timber, tone, and volume of your voice; to the sound of your breathing; and to the nature of your cough (if you're coughing).
- **Feeling:** She'll check your body temperature and assess your pulses. (In Traditional Chinese Medicine, we consult more than one pulse, and we do more than count the beats. We assess the quality of each pulse: Weak or strong? Wiry or smooth? Rising or sinking?) Your practitioner may also palpate certain areas to ascertain the exact nature of an ache or pain.

All of these observations are woven together into a diagnosis that describes a specific pattern of disharmony within your body—perhaps one that sounds more like a meteorologist's forecast (warm with a chance of showers?) than what you'd hear in a Western doctor's office.

Like meteorologists, who look at patterns of high and low pressure (not just at whether it's raining) to give their weather reports, practitioners of Traditional Chinese Medicine have their own way of defining your internal weather. They assess your health according to what we call the Eight Principles of Traditional Chinese Medicine.

- **Hot:** Characterized by activity or warmth.
- **Cold:** Characterized by lack of motion or coolness/lack of heat.
- **Interior:** Manifesting in the body's internal components (organs, brain, spinal cord, deep vessels and nerves, bones).
- **Exterior:** On the surface of the body (skin, hair, nails, capillaries and superficial nerves, nose, mouth, teeth).
- **Excessive:** Too much of a good thing; for example, too warm.
- **Deficient:** Not enough of a good thing; for example, the entire body or a specific organ does not have enough vital energy to perform its functions.
- **Yin:** Conditions that are cool, interior, and/or deficient.
- **Yang:** Conditions that are warm, exterior, and/or excessive.

It's important to note that, in making a diagnosis, an Eastern practitioner considers things most Western physicians don't take into account, such as your emotions. A practitioner of Traditional Chinese Medicine will note if you are feeling angry, sad, fearful, or worried—each an indicator of a different kind of disharmonious weather.

An Eastern practitioner will also pay attention to your body's "essences." Although there are several essences critical to our health—some familiar to us (phlegm, semen), some not (*Jing,* the primordial energy that passes to us at conception; and *Shen,* our spiritual and creative energy)—we will focus on the two that are most important to fertility: *Qi,* the life-force energy of all things; and *Blood,* the fluid that nourishes every aspect of our bodies.

QI

Qi (pronounced "chee") is the body's most dynamic, immediate energy. It animates all things, and it is everywhere—in animals and plants, in oceans and rivers, in the food we eat, in the pulsation of the cosmos itself.

FEEL YOUR QI

Having trouble grasping the concept of Qi, something omnipresent yet invisible? Try this simple exercise:

- If your hands are cool, bring warmth and Qi to them by rubbing them together briefly.
- Relax your hands and hold them in front of your upper body, forearms at elbow level. Now move your hands together until they are very close to each other but not touching. Your fingers should curve gently in as if you're holding a round object between your hands. Can you feel the energy, the Qi?
- Imagine that you are holding a ball of Qi. Now slowly move your hands apart, then back together again, taking care that your hands don't touch each other. Can you feel your Qi ball expand and contract between your palms?

Qi supports growth, change, and transformation. It takes countless forms. It enables us to maintain the structure of our bodies. It protects us, and it keeps us warm.

Some of us are blessed with strong, healthy Qi. Others, through either our physical inheritance or our lifestyles, have weaker or compromised Qi. The good news is that Qi can be transformed. For example, the Qi of illness can be changed into healthy Qi through medicine, meditation, and exercise. And although we cannot change the Qi we are born with (called *Prenatal Qi*), we can improve our overall Qi through the foods and beverages we consume and the air we breathe. (That's why our *Fertility Wisdom* includes advice on eating, drinking, and even breathing.)

Qi flows through our bodies along invisible pathways called *meridians*. There are 14 regular and 8 "extraordinary," or special, meridians that run along the surface of the body and through internal organs and tissues; a different organ governs each meridian. (If you're interested inlearning more about the body's meridians, you'll find meridian maps in *The Web That Has No Weaver*, by Ted Kaptchuk, OMD.) Connections among the meridians ensure that Qi flows evenly throughout our bodies. However, Qi can be hampered—by injury, suppressed emotions, unhealthy lifestyles, or invaders (for example, viruses). When the flow of Qi is inhibited, or when our ability to access Qi from the world around us is impaired, bad weather, disharmony, and illness occur.

BLOOD

Think back to our discussion of Yin and Yang in the previous chapter, and you'll recall that Yang is activating, dynamic, the energy of initiation—just like Qi. Yin, in contrast, is responsive, nurturing, receptive. From an Eastern perspective, these are the very qualities of Blood.

As it circulates, propelled by the Qi of our hearts, Blood moistens and nourishes our bodies. Through its constant motion, it ensures that we remain vital, not stagnant, by feeding the organs that create and control Qi.

Because Blood plays such an important role in our health, it is critical that we keep our Blood healthy. We can do this, in part, through the foods we eat—as you'll learn, a healthful diet is an important tool in enhancing Blood's contribution to fertility.

AN EASTERN APPROACH TO INFERTILITY: DISHARMONIES OF BLOOD AND QI

Men and women who are challenged by infertility often have certain physical conditions in common. Western medicine looks at these similarities in terms of allopathic diagnosis. For example, your infertility may be the result of high FSH, poor egg quality, thin uterine lining, blocked Fallopian tubes, ovarian cysts, endometriosis, irregular periods, low sperm count or motility—or it might be unexplainable from a Western perspective because, as far as Western medicine can see, there's nothing to prevent you from conceiving or carrying a baby to full term.

As you might imagine, Traditional Chinese Medicine takes a different approach to defining infertility, based on the idea of whole-person health.

Instead of looking at conditions related strictly to your reproductive organs, Eastern medicine looks at the manifestation of illness across the entire person: body and emotions; external symptoms and internal weather; the health of Blood and Qi; balance between Yin and Yang; congruency among Head, Heart, and Gut; and harmony or disharmony among the Five Elements.

Because Traditional Chinese Medicine looks at a broader array of symptoms and patterns, practitioners see different commonalities among infertile couples than Western practitioners do. It's not uncommon for three women with the same diagnosis from a Western fertility expert—say, high FSH or unexplained infertility—to have different Eastern diagnoses. Likewise, three women with the same Eastern diagnosis might have three different Western-defined fertility challenges.

In my more than 30 years of practicing Traditional Chinese Medicine— particularly my last 20 years specializing in fertility enhancement—I've learned to quickly recognize common fertility-impairing "weather reports" among men and women, regardless of their Western diagnoses. In women, fertility challenges result from disharmonies of the Blood—not surprising, since Blood is the Yin or female counterpart to Qi's Yang. In men battling infertility, common problems are related to Qi.

BLOOD DISHARMONY IN WOMEN

In Traditional Chinese Medicine there are three organs that affect how Blood functions in the body. The *Heart* powers blood circulation. The *Liver* stores Blood. And the *Spleen* governs the vessels that transport Blood throughout the body. In women, when any one of these organs is compromised, Blood may be out of harmony and fertility impaired.

There are three ways Blood can be out of harmony:

- It can be *deficient*—meaning there's not enough Blood for the organ to perform its functions.
- It can be *stagnant*—meaning that instead of flowing smoothly through your body, Blood is congealed in certain organs.
- It can be *overheated*—much like a car with low radiator fluid.

We can have the biggest impact on Blood disharmonies by altering our intake of the substances from which Blood is derived: food and drink. In Part 2, we'll explore how women can change their internal weather by changing what and how they eat and drink; by practicing a few simple acupressure, meditation, and exercise techniques; and by breathing in harmony with nature.

QI DISHARMONY IN MEN

Patterns of disharmony related to infertility in men are matters of Qi—either whole-body Qi or the Qi of organs related to fertility. These organs are the *Lungs,* which are very important as the source of protective Qi that supports the immune system, and the *Kidneys,* which, in Traditional Chinese Medicine, are related to the reproductive organs.

Most men with Qi disharmony experience Deficient Qi or even Collapsed Qi—when Qi is so deficient it can't maintain the body's structure. Some men experience Stagnant Qi or Rebellious Qi—when Qi moves in the wrong direction (such as when you cough, hiccup, vomit, or have high blood pressure).

Qi disharmonies, in which the active Yang nature of healthy Qi is compromised, are best remedied through physical activities. Men whose Qi is in disharmony can change their internal weather through exercise, acupressure, breathing techniques, meditation, or rest. You'll find information on these techniques in Part 2.

COMMON WESTERN INFERTILITY DIAGNOSES—AND THE HOPE OF TRADITIONAL CHINESE MEDICINE

Although Traditional Chinese Medicine takes its own approach to fertility issues, in our clinic we pay close attention to clients' Western fertility diagnoses and often work with Western doctors to help infertile couples conceive.

The majority of the fertility clients we see face one of the following challenges. Perhaps you do, too.

UNEXPLAINED INFERTILITY

Roughly 40 percent of fertility clients come to our clinic with a diagnosis of unexplained infertility—meaning their Western doctors can find no physical reason for their inability to conceive. These are women whose blood work shows normal hormone levels; women with normal uterine linings and no detected scar tissue, ovarian cysts, or fibroids; women whose youth and seemingly healthy eggs should produce healthy babies; women whose partners have healthy sperm. But for some reason, these women are unable to conceive—perhaps after years of trying.

Often the frustration of such a diagnosis becomes a health issue in itself: Stressed from the constant pressures of finely planned procreation—tracking cycles, taking temperatures, scheduling sexual activity—and watching every month with no sign of a baby, these women and their partners are often fatigued, depleted, discouraged, anxious, or depressed, and in no emotional state to conceive.

Although women with unexplained infertility receive identically frustrating Western diagnoses, they may display very different constitutions from a Traditional Chinese Medicine perspective. Some have internal landscapes too cool for conception; others run on the warm side. Clients at both ends of the spectrum, from cooler internal weather to warmer, have responded well to the guidelines presented in this book. So if you've received a diagnosis of "unexplained infertility" from your Western doctor, don't despair. By considering your body's deepest patterns—not just the most obvious signs of reproductive health—you can balance and harmonize your constitution and increase your chances of conceiving.

UNDIAGNOSED MALE INFERTILITY

Although we clearly recognize that creating a baby takes two—female and male, Yin and Yang—most often it's women who initiate fertility treatment. Often, too, women assume that the obstacle to conception resides in their own bodies—and often it does. But before proceeding with fertility treatment through our clinic, I always ask a female client if her male partner has been tested to rule out potential problems with his contribution to the fertility equation.

The following case illustrates why: Marilyn and her husband, Todd, were young and healthy, with no apparent barrier between them and a family. But despite the appearances of good health, they had been unable to conceive. Following the path of friends who'd used Traditional Chinese Medicine to have their baby, Marilyn and Todd came to our clinic for support. As I always do, I asked if both had considered Western medical tests to assess their fertility. Todd replied that he had not had his sperm tested but felt certain that there was "nothing wrong." Despite my encouragement, he declined to pursue testing.

Accepting her husband's decision, Marilyn embraced our *Fertility Wisdom* and submitted to treatment after treatment. Exasperated, we both finally managed to persuade Todd to consult a specialist. When he did, doctors found Todd was producing virtually no viable sperm—strong evidence that, before we invest time, energy, and resources in enhancing a woman's fertility, we must remember that conception is a two-person enterprise.

If you're a man who's been diagnosed with a sperm disorder (or a woman concerned for her male partner), you are not without resources. Men with low sperm counts, low sperm motility, reversed vasectomies, and other male reproductive challenges have successfully used the tools in this book to shift their constitutions and improve the health of their sperm. Meanwhile, women whose partners experience fertility challenges can improve the chances of bringing a baby into the family by ensuring that their own bodies are balanced, harmonized, and receptive to their partner's gift.

FIRST-TRIMESTER MISCARRIAGE

For many of the women I see, getting pregnant is no problem. Staying pregnant is. In fact, statistics show that roughly 20 percent of pregnancies end in first-trimester miscarriages. And as you know if you've experienced a miscarriage after struggling to become pregnant, losing a baby during the first trimester can be even more devastating than failing to get pregnant in the first place.

When I listen to clients talk about their miscarriages, a familiar pattern emerges: Western doctors who specialize in treating infertility focus on conception; when it occurs, they urge the happy moms to go out and live their lives. And that's exactly what these women do. They jog, bike, take intensive yoga classes. They spend hours on their feet or in front of the computer or on the phone, and they think little of traveling long distances to get where they want to go.

But the lives we live before we conceive—often hectic, self-focused, scheduled from dawn to dusk—may not be lives that nurture a struggling seed, which needs calm, quiet, consistent conditions to take root. Many hopeful parents need lifestyle coaching in order to adapt to pregnancy. They must learn to compromise (temporarily) the life they know in order to sustain the new life they've worked so hard to attract.

Yes, it can be inconvenient to avoid first-trimester travel, cut back on work, get extra sleep, avoid emotionally disruptive situations, or curtail the intense athletic activities that shape our lives and bodies. But as women who've followed our program successfully after multiple miscarriages will tell you, a gentle, centered life that includes plenty of restful sleep (and no disruptive exercise or travel) can make the difference between staying pregnant and just getting pregnant.

HIGH FSH (FOLLICLE-STIMULATING HORMONE)

FSH, measured through a blood test, is one indicator of a woman's capacity for pregnancy. Western doctors often rely on FSH tests to estimate egg quantity (called ovarian reserve) and the chance of conceiving: The higher the FSH, the lower the chances, they say.* But FSH isn't the only factor that

*Checked on the third day of the menstrual cycle, FSH should be no higher than 8 for the greatest chances of conception, many doctors say. However, one client at our clinic conceived naturally with an FSH reading of 65, and conceived her second child—again, naturally—when her FSH was 56. Both children are healthy and growing.

determines fertility, and as I've discovered through my practice, a high FSH reading often leaves women with a sense of hopelessness rather than serving as a tool for improving their chances of conception.

All too often, women come into our clinic assuming that high FSH dooms them to intensive hormone therapy, intrauterine insemination, in vitro fertilization, donor eggs, or adoption. But, when they follow my program carefully, I've seen women who, at the outset of our work together, had FSH levels higher than 100 reduce their FSH (in one case, from 118 to 9) and conceive naturally. As they prepare their bodies for pregnancy, these women stay optimistic, committed, and focused on the good work they're doing to enhance their pregnancy odds—not on one number that limits their opportunities.

AGE

In addition to FSH, Western doctors consider a woman's age when assessing the potential for conception. Countless clients, from their late thirties through their late forties, come into our clinic reporting that their doctors, based on age alone, recommend they immediately prepare for in vitro fertilization if they hope to conceive—or that they consider alternatives to having their own genetic child.

Based on their doctor's reaction, women often assume that age automatically means poor egg quality. But as many clients and I have discovered, just as a young woman will not necessarily have viable eggs, an older woman will not necessarily have eggs incapable of supporting conception. The greatest indicator of fertility, we've found, is not chronological age, but whole-person constitution and internal weather, which can be greatly improved by a woman truly committed to putting the wisdom of Traditional Chinese Medicine into practice.

THIN OR THICK UTERINE LINING

The lining of the uterus is like the soil in a garden: For a seed to sprout, the medium in which it is growing must be healthy enough to support strong roots. When a woman's endometrial lining is too thin—a common problem—or too thick, it can be difficult for an embryo to implant in the uterus. (Generally, a lining between 8 and 13 millimeters, measured by ultrasound during the time in a woman's cycle when the lining is at its thickest, is considered optimal; anything thinner than 6 millimeters or thicker than 15 millimeters may jeopardize pregnancy.)

In Traditional Chinese Medicine, we view the thickness of the endometrial lining as a reflection of the health of a woman's Blood. If her constitution is too warm or too cool, resulting in Blood that is overheated or deficient, the condition of the uterine lining and her fertility may be compromised.

Luckily, nature gives women the chance to provide a healthy medium for conception each month, when, in the absence of an implanted embryo, the uterine lining is shed. After a woman's period, the uterine lining regenerates—and if we can improve the quality of her Blood, warming or cooling her constitution as appropriate by adjusting what she eats and drinks and nurturing her body in other ways, we can increase her chances of conceiving and carrying a baby full term.

FIBROIDS, OVARIAN CYSTS, ENDOMETRIOSIS, AND SCAR TISSUE

From a Traditional Chinese Medicine perspective, uterine fibroids, ovarian cysts, endometriosis, and scar tissue are evidence of stagnant weather in the body. These pockets of congestion can hamper the flow of Blood to key organs and impede the flow of Qi, the body's vital energy.

Some of our clients have had surgeries to remove fibroids or dermoid cysts on their ovaries, or to combat endometriosis. These surgeries sometimes leave scar tissue that makes conception difficult—but not necessarily impossible. Sometimes, too, we help clients whose Fallopian tubes are blocked by scar tissue, or who carry large scars from previous C-sections or other abdominal surgeries even from childhood. In each case, Traditional Chinese Medicine offers a way to restore the flow of vital essences or help external scars regain some of the color and texture of normal skin—a good indicator that the organs beneath are better prepared for conception and full-term pregnancy.

CHECKING YOUR CONSTITUTION

Although a practitioner of Traditional Chinese Medicine would prescribe a course of treatment based on your particular pattern of disharmony—Blood or Qi; deficient, overheated, or stagnant—for the purposes of this program, our focus will be on your body's simplest expression of health: your internal weather report. (If you'd like to learn more about the disharmonies of Blood and Qi we see most often in women and men, please see Appendix C on page 211 of this book.)

As we proceed with our *Fertility Wisdom,* you will be able to customize your approach if you know how to read your body's weather report. For example, do you have a cooler constitution, in need of a subtle warmup, or a warmer constitution, which would benefit from gentle cooling? Is Blood or Qi stagnant in your body—a sign that you need to get these vital essences moving freely?

To take your constitution's temperature, explore "Common Weather Patterns" on page 46, checking the characteristics and conditions that best describe you. Then tally your results. In which category do you have the most symptoms—warmer, cooler, or stagnant? As you proceed, keep three things in mind.

First, realize that many of us have constitutions that display a combination of warm and cool signals. That's because, in reality, our constitutions manifest in two layers: a deeper layer, representing the internal weather we are born with; and a surface layer, displaying the impact of more immediate influences on our health (for example, what we ate yesterday, how active we've been).

Here's an example: Perhaps you were born with a tendency toward a cooler constitution; your whole life, you've noticed that your hands and feet are cold, you chill easily and crave warmth, and the body of your tongue tends to be pale. But you lead a fast-paced life that keeps you on your feet all the time, and you don't always pay attention to your body's need for healthy fuel and fluids. As a result, you also show signs of heat: thirst, a red-spotted tongue, and skin that has a tendency to break out. In addition, perhaps as a result of colds or allergies, you may be prone to sinus infections, which cause your nose to bleed.

A practitioner of Traditional Chinese Medicine is skilled at reading both deeper and surface levels of the constitution and providing more complex,

READING YOUR TONGUE

As you'll learn through the course of this book, your body contains many maps of itself in microcosm. For example, every major organ in your body can be reached through an acupuncture point in your ear, or by massaging points around your navel or on the soles of your feet. Likewise, your tongue reflects your whole-body constitution. (If you look at your tongue in a mirror, you will notice that it is shaped similarly to the trunk of your body, only upside down—head and neck at the tip, hips at the base.)

By looking at the color of your tongue, the nature of its coating (or moss), and the presence of any lines, cracks, or spots, a practitioner of Traditional Chinese Medicine can assess the nature and location of disharmonies within your body. And with a little practice, you, too, can use your tongue to check your internal weather.

Because of its relationship with the food we eat and its connection to the Spleen (through the Five Elements), the tongue is an ideal tool for checking in on the condition of the Blood in women. However, men can also check their tongues for evidence of warming or cooling trends, or of stagnation. Think of it as opening a window onto your internal garden. Stick out your tongue and look in the mirror. How is the weather today?

SYMPTOM	DIAGNOSIS	WEATHER REPORT
Pale tongue	Deficient	Cooler constitution
Red or cracked tongue, little moss*	Overheated	Warmer constitution
Purplish tongue	Stagnant	May be warm or cool. A purplish/red tongue indicates stagnation with a warmer constitution. A pale and purplish or purplish/blue tongue indicates stagnation with a cooler constitution.

*Moss is the coating that sometimes appears on the tongue. It may be white or yellowish.

customized care than we could ever recommend through a book—but that doesn't mean you can't use these guidelines to improve your own internal weather. If you show signs of both warm and cool constitutions, your goal will be to achieve balance: enough exercise *and* enough rest; and foods and beverages that support a more neutral internal environment.

In addition, it's important to keep in mind that your constitution—particularly as it manifests on the surface of your body—may change day to day, depending on the outside weather, your daily activities, your immediate environment, and the season of the year. By checking your internal weather

Your Tongue Is a Map of Your Body

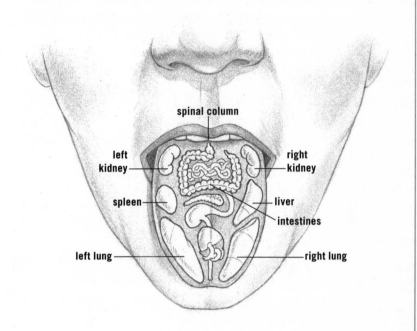

spinal column

left
kidney

right
kidney

spleen

liver

intestines

left lung

right lung

The condition of your tongue reveals the health of your body's major organs.

frequently, you can monitor changes in your constitution and adjust your fertility enhancement program to maintain balance and harmony.

Finally, be aware that a stagnant constitution may be either warm or cool. If you check many items in the Stagnant column on page 47, tally your responses in the other two columns to see if you have stagnation with a warmer constitution (for example, a purplish tongue with red spots) or stagnation with a cooler constitution (for example, uterine fibroids and a pale tongue).

If you can't tell if your constitution is cool, warm, stagnant, or some combination of these three weather patterns, don't despair. The tools presented in Part 2 of this book can be used by anyone to improve the chances of conceiving and carrying a baby. Like the apple seed that holds the potential for future fruit, you have everything you need to grow your garden. With the gifts at hand, we will work together to establish conditions that are happy, healthy, harmonious, and hopeful—the perfect weather for miracles.

COMMON WEATHER PATTERNS

You can determine your body's weather pattern by noting the following signs of warmth, coolness, and stagnation.

WARMER	COOLER	STAGNANT
• Red tongue • Red face • Skin eruptions • Thirst • Constipation • Dense menstrual flow • Warmer limbs • Restless sleep, nightmares • Prefer cooler drinks • Tendency to be more active	• Pale tongue • Pale face • Loose bowel movements • Cooler limbs • Scanty or absent menstrual flow • Need more sleep • Prefer warm drinks • Prefer less activity	• Purplish tongue • Cysts • Fibroids • Scarring • Stop-and-start menstrual flow • Purplish and/or clotted menstrual flow • Gas • Sudden mood changes • Alternate between loose stool and constipation • Sensation of fluctuating body temperature (feel hot, then feel cold)

Toby's Story

KEEPING THE PROMISE

*D*octors couldn't explain why Roberta, 40, couldn't get pregnant. She'd tried Clomid (a drug commonly used to induce ovulation, correct irregular ovulation, or help increase egg production), hormone injections, and five intrauterine insemination cycles. And she was scheduled for in vitro fertilization at one of the top fertility clinics in her home state. When her progesterone level proved too high for implantation, doctors canceled her procedure, froze the two fertilized eggs they'd planned to implant, and agreed to try again in 3 months, combining any new eggs with the frozen eggs.

Roberta and her husband, Sean, made a plan: During that 3 months, they would do everything possible to prepare Roberta's body for IVF—with luck, enabling her to produce more viable eggs. So they left their home state and came all the way to San Francisco to our clinic for help.

When Roberta opened her mouth during our intake examination, I saw signs of an extremely overheated constitution—a bright red tongue with a crack in the middle. A change in the foods and beverages she consumed would be critical to Roberta's success, as would other techniques—such as the Six Healing Sounds (see page 123)—to harmonize her internal weather and bring her body into balance.

After several treatments, Roberta and Sean returned home, committed to continuing our fertility program on their own. Changing the way Roberta nourished her body proved a challenge at first; to bring variety to her meals, she had to find new places to shop. But the efforts paid off after just 5 weeks, when Roberta experienced a breakthrough: Her period, which had almost vanished in the previous 5 years, returned with a normal, bright red flow. This success gave Roberta a huge psychological boost; for the first time in ages, she felt something positive happening in her body. She also noticed *that her complexion looked better, and she had more energy. Encouraged, she continued with the program.*

When Roberta and Sean returned to their local fertility clinic after 3 months, they ended up with three top-quality embryos to implant. The procedure went well, and soon Rebecca and Sean were back in our clinic for a follow-up. Although she was afraid to believe the procedure had been successful, her pulses told me she was pregnant. Shortly thereafter, a blood test confirmed the good news.

Roberta and Sean had expected to be overjoyed. But they had not anticipated that along with the joy of pregnancy would come the fear of losing the precious and vulnerable seed they'd worked so hard to plant. For the first weeks of her pregnancy, Roberta worried constantly about losing the baby, even though she had no history of miscarriage.

When Roberta came back to our clinic in her 7th week of pregnancy, she shared her worries, and I discovered that her emotional condition, from an Eastern perspective, betrayed cause for concern. Since becoming pregnant, Roberta had all but abandoned our program, from the eating and drinking guidelines to the breathing exercises to the herbs I had prescribed—and her body could tell the difference. What's more, her pulses indicated not just one implanted embryo, but the possibility of two.

I told Roberta of my concerns—and about the second embryo—and urged her, for her baby's sake, to maintain her commitment to balance and harmony throughout her pregnancy. But she'd just had an ultrasound the day before, and the implanted embryo—just one—looked fine, she said. There was no reason, Roberta tried to convince herself as well as me, to worry.

The next day, Roberta awoke to bleeding and cramps, just as if she were beginning her period. She panicked and immediately went in for another ultrasound. To their great relief, she and Sean discovered that their baby was fine—but that Roberta had been carrying a second embryo that had implanted but failed to thrive. Now her body was shedding it.

That day, Roberta told me, she learned three important lessons: She learned to listen to Dr. Wu. More important, she learned to listen to her own body. And most important of all, she learned to keep her promises. After all, Roberta had first attracted a baby spirit by making her body a harmonious place to grow. By recommitting herself to maintaining good internal weather throughout her pregnancy—and re-embracing the wisdom of Quan Yin—she kept the first commitment she ever made to Toby, the baby boy whose bright promise is now her pride and joy.

CHAPTER 3

ARE YOU READY FOR YOUR BABY?

As you've already learned, pursuing Traditional Chinese Medicine as a path toward pregnancy requires you to embrace concepts that differ dramatically from Western ways of thinking. Now I'd like to remind you of what may be another difficult new concept to grasp: *You* have no control over whether you will get pregnant and when and how your baby will arrive. It's not *you* who decides. It's your *baby*.

Although you ultimately can't control the outcome of your efforts to conceive, you can do something very powerful: You can send an invitation by making your body a welcome place for new life to grow. Your physical health, your mental state, your emotional outlook, your lifestyle, your relationships—all send signals about your pregnancy readiness to the child you hope to attract and (even more important) carry full-term. Sending a welcoming message may require you to make challenging changes in your health and habits. It's time for you and your partner to take a long, hard look at yourselves and decide whether or not to implement the changes that will make you ready for your baby.

ATTRACTING NEW LIFE

So, what does it mean to be ready for your baby? It means that both you and your partner are fully committed to and prepared for parenting. It means that you are in harmony about how to raise your child, and that you have the physical, mental, and emotional capacity—including the patience—to be the kind of parents you want to be.

It also means that you are in balance as individuals: What you do is congruent with what you think and feel—meaning that the Heaven, Human, and Earth levels of your being are aligned, as we discussed previously. Here's an example of incongruence: If you think you're committed to your relationship yet you spend all your time at work (to your partner's chagrin), your actions (Earth brain) are out of alignment with your thoughts (Heaven brain), and perhaps your feelings (Human brain). Here's another: You think you want a baby (Heaven brain) and feel very open to loving a child (Human brain), yet you and your partner can never find the

ESTABLISHING CONGRUENCY WITH YOUR PARTNER

In chapter 2, you learned about the importance of establishing congruency within yourself, among Heaven, Human, and Earth and the elements of your being that connect you to these realms. But to create the ideal environment for new life, you must be congruent with your partner as well as within yourself. Imagine the connection you feel when the two of you breathe in sync. That kind of alignment, sustained over time, helps turn couples into potential parents.

To determine where you and your partner are already in sync and where you may be manifesting different ideas and rhythms, complete the following exercise together at a time when you have no distractions. To tap the power of the Five Elements, write your answers on colored paper or using colored pens (or pencils) as indicated:

- Without talking, take a moment to focus quietly on the prospect of pregnancy, the challenges you face in achieving your goal, and your future baby.
- Without looking at each other's answers, take a piece of green paper or a pen with green ink and respond to the following question: *What does your head (your Heaven brain) want?*
- Now take a piece of pink or red paper or a pink or red pen and answer this question: *What does your heart (your Human brain) want?*

time to make love while you're most fertile (Earth brain). To maximize your potential for conception, it's important that you explore any think-feel-do incongruences and the impact they might have on your readiness for parenting.

When couples come to my clinic for help with fertility, I ask them a series of questions about their physical, emotional, and spiritual health. These question-and-answer sessions help us identify any stumbling blocks to conception and carrying a child to term, then determine whether and how to move forward. You'll find those questions in this chapter.

Because attracting new life requires that both partners be fully aligned in their commitment, it's important that you work through these questions

---

- Take a piece of yellow paper or a yellow pen and answer this: *What does your gut (your Earth brain) have to tell you?*
- At this point, you should have three pieces of paper of three different colors or with messages written in three different colors of ink. Now take a pen of your favorite color and consolidate your answers on a single piece of white paper.

Share and discuss your responses with your partner. Where are your desires in alignment? Where do they differ? Then, complete the following steps together, using colored pens and a single piece of white paper:

- Using your Heaven brains together, talk out a reasonable solution that can bring you into alignment on issues where you differ. Write your solution in green ink on the white piece of paper.
- Using your Human brains together, discuss how you will make greater efforts to share your feelings with each other to maintain alignment. Write down your ideas in pink or red ink on the white paper.
- Using your Earth brains together, discuss the practical resources you'll need to maintain congruency between yourselves over time. Add your answer in yellow ink to the white paper. You should now have a single piece of white paper that integrates the best "thinking" of your Heaven, Human, and Earth brains.

TALKING WITH YOUR PARTNER

Depending on how well you and your partner communicate, you may find the questions in this chapter difficult to discuss. If you feel daunted by the challenge, remember that getting these issues out in the open now is critical—not only to attracting new life, but also to ensuring that your child is healthy and loved.

Here are some tips for making your conversation more comfortable:

- Set aside quiet time to talk through the questions—no television, telephone, or other distractions not while driving.
- Don't try to answer all of the questions at once. Work through one section at a time. And take breaks if you're feeling overwhelmed.
- Set aside preconceived notions; be open to your partner's ideas.
- Don't overreact if you disagree. Take time to listen—and hold off on your response until you fully understand your partner's message.
- Once you are ready to respond, approach your differences from the standpoint of compromise rather than trying to prove your point.
- Be aware of any tendencies either of you have toward guilt, blame, and emotional hurt during these discussions. These tendencies may indicate that you would benefit from a counselor before bringing a child into the world.

together—truthfully and without distractions. When you're finished, don't look for an answer key; you won't find a scoring mechanism that indicates to what degree you're ready to be a parent, or a checklist telling you exactly what to do if you're not ready. Our goal is to empower you with information, and let you decide what to do with it.

WHERE DO YOU GO FROM HERE?

Ideally, you'll answer the questions in this chapter and discover that you're already sending out a compelling invitation—that both you and your partner are ready for conception in body, mind, and spirit, and that you're in alignment about what it means to be parents. In that case, the practices offered in this book will help you send an even stronger signal of readiness to your baby.

In reality, however, I find that many prospective parents must confront a few issues before they're truly prepared for parenthood. And, in some cases, the issues are greater than the couples want to address. In fact, some couples have decided not to continue with fertility treatment as a result of these discussions.

But many others have emerged from our question-and-answer sessions more committed than ever. They've diligently followed our *Fertility Wisdom* to work through their personal challenges to conception. They've resolved compatibility issues to create a more harmonious, welcoming environment for new life. And many of those couples have conceived, despite seemingly insurmountable odds.

As you proceed with your own self-discovery process, remember one thing: I am your coach in this effort, but not your judge. Only you can answer these questions fully and honestly and decide where you go from here. If you choose to move forward, we will work together to make your invitation to new life as compelling as it can be—and to give you the best possible chance of carrying that life to full term.

 IF YOUR FAMILY IS NONTRADITIONAL

In my clinical practice, I've worked with all kinds of couples, including those in which both partners are female. Whether your parenting partner is male or female, you'll find that the family- and relationship-related questions in our questionnaire provide plenty of food for thought, planning, and deeper partnership.

It's also possible for a single woman to embrace our *Fertility Wisdom* and conceive a child. If you don't have a partner, answer the questions in this chapter on your own. In addition, consider this: To whom will you turn for physical, financial, and emotional support if and when you need it? If possible, work through the questions in the Relationship and Level of Commitment sections with potential supporters. In so doing, you'll find out if you can count on these resources for the help you may very well need to welcome and raise your baby.

DR. WU'S FERTILITY READINESS QUESTIONNAIRE

Are you and your partner prepared to embark on the journey toward *Fertility Wisdom*? The following questions will help you assess your readiness. Some questions apply to men and women alike; others are tailored to men or women.

I recommend that both partners spend time considering these questions privately; perhaps you'll want to jot down your answers. Then, when both partners have completed the questionnaire, dedicate time to talking through your answers together. You may learn things about each other that you didn't know—things that will make pregnancy, childbirth, and child-rearing a more positive partnership endeavor. For suggestions on how to assess your responses and formulate your next steps, see "Summing It All Up" on page 63.

GENERAL HEALTH

Your medical history can have a major impact on your ability to conceive. If you or your partner has a serious medical condition, think about whether you are willing and able to address it. If you don't address your health issues now, will you truly have the strength and ability to care for a child?

1. Do you have any chronic medical conditions—obesity, underweight, diabetes, heart disease, cancer or precancerous conditions, organ disease, addictions? What can you do to control these conditions before, during, and after pregnancy (e.g., working with your doctor regarding diet and exercise, or consulting a specialist regarding the impact of these conditions on pregnancy)?

2. How is your energy? Do you feel vital and able to sustain physical activity throughout the day? Or are you weak and tired? If your energy is low, do you know of any underlying health conditions that might be the cause? What can you do to address them? If underlying health conditions are not the issue, are you getting enough rest? Can you make more time for sleep at night and naps or quiet time during

the day? And what lifestyle issues do you need to address to improve your energy (e.g., eating junk food, drinking coffee, skipping breakfast, not exercising enough—or exercising too much, an issue for many of the women I see in my clinic)?

3. Are you able to relax when you want or need to? Or are you tense and unable to let go of stress? What relaxation techniques can you integrate into your life (e.g., exercise, meditation, taking time for yourself)?

REPRODUCTIVE HEALTH

Traditional Chinese Medicine pays close attention to the many manifestations of health, including the essences that make up or emanate from our bodies. Creating a healthy baby requires the combination of healthy female and male essences (menstrual blood and semen). To ensure healthy essences, the liver, heart, spleen, lungs, and kidneys must be in harmony. Poor eating and drinking habits, lack of rest, stress, overwhelming or denied emotions, and lack of exercise can all have a negative impact on these organs and the essences they produce.

To assess your pregnancy readiness, take a close look at the reproductive histories of both your partner and yourself and observe your essences. If your answers to these questions suggest that your reproductive system or your partner's is out of harmony, you'll find self-healing practices throughout this book to help you restore health and balance.

1. Do you have/have you had sexually transmitted diseases (STDs) or infections? Have you sought treatment and consulted your doctor to see if there will be any impact on your long-term reproductive health?

2. Have you had operations on your reproductive organs? If so, have you consulted your doctor to see if there will be any impact on your long-term reproductive health? If so, have you taken any possible steps to remedy the repercussions of previous surgery?

3. Have you had difficulties with conception in the past? If so, do you

understand the source of these difficulties (e.g., physical or emotional)?

4. Have you had children before? If so, how many and when? Be aware that, for the fertility-challenged, conceiving the second time can be more difficult. Often, new mothers are preoccupied with their babies and do not take care of themselves, which can compromise their health over the long term. Have you taken time to care for your body since your earlier pregnancy? Have you resolved any emotional or practical issues and questions related to the impact of an additional child on your family?

5. Have you used fertility treatments in the past? What were the results? If you weren't successful, do you understand why?

6. Do you have a family history of unhealthy genetic patterns or diseases related to reproductive health? Have you taken steps to understand and/or remedy the condition? How have others in your family addressed this condition?

WOMEN

1. Do your periods come at regular intervals? Do you have a healthy menstrual flow (bright red blood that is free from clotting; moderate flow—3 to 4 days; little to no cramping, premenstrual breast distention, or PMS)? If not, have you consulted your doctor and/or a nutritionist about this? Are there any underlying health issues that you need to address?

2. What birth control methods have you used? Have they had any impact on your reproductive health? For example, if you've taken birth control pills, how long has it been since you stopped? Have you allowed enough time for your body to get back to its natural rhythm?

3. If you've been pregnant before, have you miscarried or had childbirth complications? Do you understand the source of these complications? Has your doctor identified any long-term repercussions?

4. Have you had an abortion in the past? If so, have you dealt with the emotional impact of this action? Are you carrying any feelings that may affect your ability to conceive again?

5. Are you aware of when you ovulate? (Over-the-counter ovulation kits are not the most reliable way to predict ovulation. For a more certain way to pinpoint the days when you are most fertile, I recommend the book Taking Charge of Your Fertility by Toni Weschler, referenced in Appendix A on page 201 of this book.)

6. What has your Western doctor told you about why you have been unable to conceive? Have you had your hormone levels (FSH/LH) tested? Has your doctor evaluated the thickness of your uterine lining?

MEN

1. Do you have any problems with erection or ejaculation? If so, have you consulted your doctor to determine the possible cause?

2. Does your semen appear healthy (white, heavy, sweet, plentiful)? If not, have you consulted your doctor and/or a nutritionist to see if there are any underlying health issues?

3. Have you had your sperm analyzed? If so, what did the analysis reveal that may affect your chances of conception?

LIFESTYLE

How you treat your own body before, during, and after pregnancy can affect your ability to conceive, as well as your child's long-term health. If your answers to the preceding questions reveal challenges related to reproductive health, your lifestyle might be a contributing factor. Changing the way you live, eat, and drink can improve egg quality or other factors related to fertility if you're a woman, or improve the quantity, quality, and vitality of your sperm if you're a man. Are you willing to do what it takes?

1. Do you consume coffee, alcoholic beverages, junk food, sugar, or cold and iced foods and drinks? Are you undernourished—perhaps because you tend to skip meals? Are you willing to change your eating and drinking habits?

2. Do you have any addictions—for example, cigarettes, alcohol, painkillers? Are you willing to eliminate these habits?

3. What are your exercise patterns? Do you need to be more physically active, or is exercise (perhaps too much of it) part of your everyday life? Are you willing to commit to a healthy exercise program? (Depending on your constitution, this might mean adding more activity to your day, or it could mean cutting back on vigorous exercise.)
4. Do you get enough sleep?
5. Do you dress warmly in cooler weather?
6. Are you exposed through your job, hobbies, or environment to chemicals, loud noises, toxins, radiation, gases, extreme temperatures, or safety hazards? Are you willing to change jobs, give up hobbies, or relocate to provide a safe environment for you and your child?

EMOTIONAL/SPIRITUAL HEALTH

Overwhelming or denied emotions such as worry, anxiety, fear, or anger can have a detrimental effect on your reproductive health, an unborn child's attraction to you as a parent, and—if you have a baby—your child's psychological health. If you or your partner has issues in this area, are you willing to confront them? Are you willing to enhance your spiritual health as well?

1. What kind of relationship did/do you have with your parents? Do you have emotional issues that might affect your ability to love and care for a child? Have you done everything possible to address these issues before moving forward with a family of your own?
2. Have you ever been in an abusive relationship? If so, how might this affect your ability to be a parent? Have you sought the help you might need to overcome these obstacles to your own happy family?
3. Do you experience excessive worry, fear, anxiety, or anger? Have you identified the source of these feelings and explored therapy or stress reduction tools to manage them?
4. Can you express emotion in a healthy way? If not, have you identified the source of this problem and explored therapy or other emotional support systems to address it?

5. Do you take time for yourself each day (through meditation, prayer, journaling, or some other form of relaxation)? Are you willing to make reflection and relaxation a regular part of your life?
6. Does your life have a satisfying spiritual component? Are you willing to commit to a spiritual practice to enhance your well-being?
7. What positive tools have you developed in your life to help yourself at difficult times? How can you apply those tools now to create a happier, more harmonious life?

RELATIONSHIP

In Traditional Chinese Medicine, we believe a child can sense emotional discord long before birth. Ideally, you and your partner should be in harmony and equipped with healthy ways to work through differences. If you aren't, having a baby will only add to your conflicts. If you face problems in your relationship, are you willing to get help from a counselor to create a more harmonious environment for your child?

1. How long have you been married or committed to each other?
2. Are you emotionally connected in a positive way?
3. How well do you and your partner communicate? Do you work through disagreements without guilt, blame, and emotional hurt?
4. Do you respect each other's point of view?
5. If your answers to these questions reveal difficulties in your relationship, have you and your partner attempted to address these issues together? Have you sought support from a couples counselor or therapist? What steps are you willing to take to improve your relationship before you add a child to it?

LEVEL OF COMMITMENT

Many couples rush headlong into pregnancy without considering why and whether they truly want a child. Are you ready to raise a child? Do you have a plan for how you will take care of the new life you bring into this world?

If you and your partner have fundamental differences about these issues, take the time to discuss them thoroughly. Recognize that these differences place you at a disadvantage in conceiving and in how your lives will be if you have a child. Think through the following questions carefully and answer as honestly as you can.

1. Why do you want a baby?
2. Are you 100 percent committed to being a parent?
3. How do you and your partner define family? Are your definitions compatible?
4. Do you feel confident about your ability to be a parent? Why or why not?
5. How do you expect your lifestyle will change once you have a child?
6. Do you have the energy, focus, and capacity to care for a child?
7. Do you have concerns about giving up your free time, hobbies, career, or financial comfort in order to care for your child?
8. What are your work hours? Are you willing to cut back on your work or even change your profession in order to spend enough time with your child?
9. Are you willing to sacrifice social activities and hobbies in order to spend enough time with your child?
10. Do you and your partner hold the same beliefs and philosophies about how to raise a child?
11. Will you be able to love a child during stressful conditions such as sleep deprivation, financial challenges, work deadlines, or your partner's unavailability?
12. Do you have the financial resources to provide a safe and healthy environment for your child?
13. Are you willing to rethink your personal, financial, and business goals in order to provide the support your child will need?
14. Are you willing to make changes to your home or even move so that you can provide enough space and a healthy environment for your child?

15. If your answers to these questions reveal conflict between you and your partner, what are you willing to do to work through these issues (e.g., couples counseling, therapy, delaying pregnancy until you and your spouse are in sync)?

SUMMING IT ALL UP

Now that you've run my gauntlet of tough questions, take a moment to assess your answers and prepare yourself for your next steps by completing the following exercise. Do this exercise with your partner, writing down your answers to the six questions that follow. Then reinforce your commitment by following steps seven and eight.

1. What strengths do your answers to the questions in this chapter reveal?

2. In what areas do your major challenges lie: general or reproductive health? lifestyle? emotional/spiritual health? relationship? level of commitment?

3. What changes do you feel you must make in order to welcome new life?

4. Which of these changes will be easiest to make? Which will be most challenging?

5. If you were to summarize your next steps in the form of a strategy, what would that strategy be? Try completing the following sentence: *To make my body a welcoming place for new life, I will . . .* (Examples: *Start a healthy exercise regimen to get in better physical shape before attempting to conceive. Track my menstrual cycles more carefully to observe patterns before attempting to conceive. Give up coffee. Commit to couples counseling to address communications challenges. Pay greater attention to my spiritual health. Commit myself to fully exploring Fertility Wisdom.*).

6. Identify people to whom you can turn for support when following through on your strategy. How will you engage these family members, friends, and supporters in your plans from the beginning?

7. Using the meditation exercise on page 10, form a clear picture—one you and your partner agree upon—of what success will look like. Write down every detail. Use this description to remind yourself of what's at stake if ever you lose sight of your goal.

8. We've talked about how important it is to send your future baby positive, welcoming signals. But what about the messages your mind is sending your body? If you've struggled to conceive, you may find that many discouraging messages echo in your head—"I'll never get pregnant." "Doctors say it's impossible." "I can't face another failed pregnancy attempt." Or, past behaviors such as an abortion or sexual promiscuity can engender thoughts of guilt—"I made a terrible mistake." "I can't get pregnant because I'm being punished." These messages can affect your emotional state and your physical health. Right now, start sending yourself positive messages by embracing this affirmation: *My body welcomes new life.* Write it down, and remember it.

Zoe and Zach's Story
REDEFINING "REGULAR"

*T*ina's periods had never been "regular" by Western medicine's usual definition. Instead of menstruating every 28 or 30 days, her periods came roughly every 40 days. And in a woman of 50 years, doctors told her, such "irregularity" meant one thing: the onset of menopause.

Although she'd already raised children from another marriage 20 years earlier, Tina wasn't ready to give up on having a baby with her current husband, Craig. In search of a hopeful alternative to her Western diagnosis, she came to our clinic.

Tina's case illustrates what we often see in women who are approaching what Western medicine perceives as their reproductive *sunset. Because Traditional Chinese Medicine looks at internal weather—not chronological age—I was able to give Tina a more hopeful prognosis: By balancing and harmonizing her overheated, dry, stagnant constitution—and calming her busy life—we could create an environment conducive to conception, regardless of her age.*

Tina embraced our program with the same dedication she'd applied in her former career as a professional dancer and in her current life as the manager of a big hotel restaurant. And she took my advice on one more thing: Instead of viewing fertility enhancement as her personal project, she engaged Craig in the program—explaining what she was doing, including him in decisions, strengthening their partnership. Their shared dedication to fertility and its gifts came in handy when their twins, Zoe and Zach—conceived naturally—arrived, turning hopeful couple into happy family.

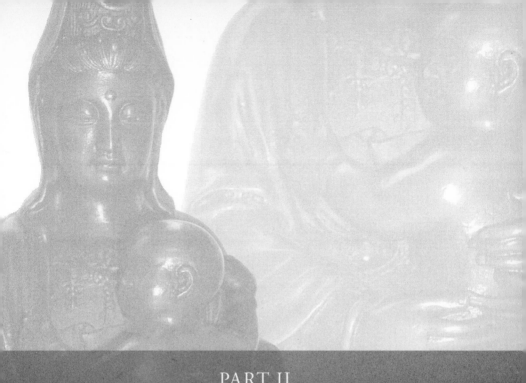

PART II

BALANCING AND HARMONIZING, STEP BY STEP

You've explored the wisdom of the Tao and examined how Traditional Chinese Medicine views infertility. You've taken a step back to consider the signals your physical, emotional, and spiritual health are sending your future baby. And you and your partner have committed to doing what it takes to attract new life.

Now it's time for you to move out of theory and into action by following our *Fertility Wisdom* program step by step, so that you can achieve balance, harmony, and congruency—the ideal conditions for conceiving and carrying your miracle baby.

Before we begin, let me offer a word of advice: *Be patient.* Preparing your body for conception doesn't happen overnight. It takes time to come into balance after years of habits that may not have served you well. So, be certain your expectations are realistic.

Please prepare yourself to follow this program diligently for at least 3 to 6 months before trying to conceive—then another 3 to 6 months before assessing your results.

CONNECTING WITH THE ENERGY OF QUAN YIN

As we discussed in the Introduction, Quan Yin, the original Chinese fertility goddess, offers the gift of new life. To accept her gift, we must get in touch with our bodies: how it feels to inhabit them and what they need to thrive.

What better way to do this than through things we do every day: eat, drink, breathe, and move—the activities we'll explore in Part II? As we discussed in chapter 2, when we looked at possible causes of infertility from an Eastern perspective, these activities have a dramatic impact on the internal weather that makes your body either a hospitable place or a hostile climate. Indeed, the tools to change your body are right here in your hands, and you are about to put those hands to work.

FIRST THINGS FIRST: SOME PRACTICAL WISDOM

Western and Eastern cultures alike regard elders as a source of knowledge on how to live a healthy life. And many of these wise elders are women. Who among us hasn't had a grandmother or a mother or a great aunt who, whether we requested it or not, offered us advice about living right? ("Don't go swimming right after a meal!" "Zip up your jacket or you'll catch your death of cold!") And how often have we ignored such practical advice as nothing more than quaint folk wisdom?

The truth is, there's *real* wisdom in some of these practical cautions. And in China, such grandmotherly advice—like my grandmother's poached egg recipe (see page 72)—often reflects the most basic concepts of Traditional Chinese Medicine.

For example, China is full of concerned grandmothers who tell their busy granddaughters never to leave the house with wet hair—or, for that matter, not to wash their hair at all during their periods. Many modern Chinese women, as their Western counterparts would, brush off such advice and hurry out the door. But the truth is, from a Traditional Chinese Medicine perspective, running around outside with a mop of wet hair—particularly in cold weather, or when your body is already experiencing internal dampness (i.e., during your period)—is like inviting damp weather to inhabit your head. Ignore your Chinese grandmother and, over time, you may find yourself with a dampness disharmony, which might present itself as headaches or the tendency to catch colds during your period.

Here's another example: Your Chinese grandmother would shake her finger at you in disapproval if she saw you eating ice cream or sipping a glass of iced tea—especially during your period, or if you are trying to get pregnant. Why? Because putting anything iced in your body—particularly when your energies are consumed by menstruation or attempts at conception—is like inviting winter to invade your abdomen. Bite after creamy bite, slurp after frosty slurp, cold treats will turn your fertile garden into

AMA'S POST-PERIOD/POSTPARTUM POACHED CHICKEN OR EGGS

When I was a teenager living in my grandparents' house, my mother's step-mother—I never knew her real name, but I called her Ama—would insist I eat a particular breakfast every month after my period had ended completely. The more I learned about Traditional Chinese Medicine, the better I understood the science behind Ama's recommendation: Energetically, it's a recipe for vitality when the body's Qi has been depleted from menstruation or childbirth. Try it yourself, post-period or postpartum—but only after all bleeding has ceased.

However, please note: I recommend this recipe *only* if you are not trying to become pregnant right away—for example, if you're giving your body several months to strengthen itself prior to attempting conception. Why? Because, as you'll learn when we explore food energies in greater detail, poultry has a warming and constricting energy. Sesame oil, too, is warming. Once you begin trying to conceive, we'll be striving to maintain a balanced internal environment: not too warm, not too cool.

1	cup chicken broth or water
3	slices fresh gingerroot
1	teaspoon sesame oil
3	tablespoons rice wine
2	eggs or one serving chicken meat*

Bring the broth or water, ginger, sesame oil, and rice wine to a simmer. Add the eggs or chicken, plus enough water to cover if necessary. Return to a simmer and poach to desired doneness. Eat the eggs or chicken and drink the broth, discarding the ginger.

*The traditional recipe calls for chicken meat, but when I was growing up, my family could not afford chicken, so we used eggs instead.

frozen tundra. And the new life you're trying to attract and cultivate does not thrive in an Arctic climate.

So let's take a moment to thank our ancestors for their timeless advice and set a few practical, healthy ground rules that will have Quan Yin (and our grandmothers, Western and Eastern) smiling in approval.

So that Quan Yin hears your voice and may offer you her support, I would like for you to read the following commitments aloud:

While following the *Fertility Wisdom* program, I will:
- Get plenty of deep, restful sleep—at least 8 hours a night.
- Stop smoking.
- Avoid alcohol, soft drinks, and coffee.
- Replace junk food with real food.
- Give up cold and iced foods and drinks, including ice cream.
- Get regular, moderate exercise—at least an energizing walk every day.*
- Dry my hair thoroughly before leaving home.
- Dress warmly in cold weather—and always wear a hat in winter.

A TWO-PHASE APPROACH

If you've been trying to get pregnant for some time, or if you've paid close attention to your reproductive health over the years, you probably already know the length of your menstrual cycle and when you ovulate. If you don't know when you ovulate, try an over-the-counter ovulation kit, available in most drugstores. For the purposes of this program, we will divide your cycle—whether it's 28 days, 30 days, or more or less—into two phases: before you ovulate, and after you ovulate.

In my clinical practice, it's not unusual for me to recommend that a couple stop trying to conceive for at least 3 months while our *Fertility Wisdom* brings bodies into balance, congruency, and harmony. However, if you continue to try to conceive from Day 1 of this program (or even if you have intercourse without the intent of pregnancy), there will always be the possibility that you've become pregnant.

As you may know, the phase between conception—the union of

---

*Clients often ask me when is the best time to exercise. My answer: Listen to your body. If you find that exercise revs you up, schedule it to take advantage of this energizing effect—for example, in the morning. If you find that exercise calms or tires you, schedule it for later in the day, to help you unwind or prepare for sleep.

sperm and egg—and the implantation of a fertilized egg is a delicate time, during which we must treat new life (or even the potential for it) with great care. In the first half of your cycle, we will be creating a receptive, energetically balanced environment that welcomes conception. In the second half of your cycle, from the day you ovulate through the first day of your next period (if it arrives), we will be taking extra precautions to ensure that any viable, fertilized eggs have the opportunity to implant in the uterus. In other words, we will be working for the calmest, most stable internal weather possible—no cyclones, floods, freezes, or heat waves. That means avoiding emotionally upsetting situations, activities that dramatically increase heart rate and circulation (particularly to the abdomen), and anything physically taxing during this phase of your cycle.

Starting 24 hours before ovulation until Day 1 of your next menstrual cycle (or through the first trimester if you become pregnant), please avoid the following activities:

- Travel by air or by car on bumpy roads.
- Vigorous exercise—particularly anything that activates the pubococcygeus (PC) muscle, which supports the pelvic floor and surrounds the reproductive organs. (If you've ever done Kegel exercises, you understand what it means to activate the PC muscle.*) This is why I recommend refraining from Kegels between ovulation and the start of your menstrual cycle, or through the first trimester of pregnancy. The same rule applies to doing situps, riding a bicycle, and climbing stairs or slopes—all activities that activate the PC muscle and should be avoided. (If you live in a building with many stairs, of course you can't completely avoid stair climbing, but you *can* apply this PC-muscle-friendly climbing technique: Take baby steps. Put one foot up on a step, then bring your other foot up to the same step. Repeat.)
- Vigorous sexual activity. (Sexual activity is fine through the day you ovulate, but afterward you will need to avoid anything that dramatically increases bloodflow to the abdomen or stimulates uterine contractions, including deep orgasms. So be gentle!)

- Shoulder rubs. Massaging the shoulders can stimulate acupuncture points that encourage energy to move down in the body. In fact, when a practioner of Traditional Chinese Medicine seeks to induce labor, he or she needles the shoulders.
- Baths and swimming. (Short showers—neither too hot nor too cold— are acceptable.)
- Intense emotional experiences (e.g., through conversations, books, or movies).
- Spicy or pungent foods. (They add disruptive heat to your internal weather.)
- Scented products such as bath oils, essential oils, incense, candles, sachets, lotions, and perfumes. (Odors can have a powerful impact on the body. For example, some perfumes have a warm, pungent energy that causes Qi and/or Blood to disperse—something we want to prevent if you are in the early stages of pregnancy. Strong scents can also be overstimulating during pregnancy.)
- Ginger juice or dried ginger. (Often used for morning sickness, raw or dried ginger, like warm or pungent odors, has a tendency to disperse energy and should be avoided if you are pregnant. If you experience nausea, use a seasickness wristband or snack on preserved Umeboshi plums, a traditional Asian remedy for nausea in the early stages of pregnancy. Many grocery stores carry preserved plums among other Asian foods.)

If you may be pregnant, there is one action that I do encourage: Eat poultry (preferably organic). Whereas raw or dried ginger and pungent odors can disperse the energy we are trying to maintain in your abdomen, poultry has a constricting effect, which can help protect the fetus from miscarriage. (Think of it this way: At the beginning of a pregnancy, the tiny embryo is like a little chunk of blood; you want that tiny bit of blood

---

*To find out where your PC muscle is and how to activate it, try this: While urinating, squeeze the muscles in your pubic area to stop your urine flow. Now release. You've just activated your PC muscle.

IT'S IN YOUR HANDS

Through my fertility practice, I've learned that many women and men find meditation an unsettling rather than a relaxing or enlightening practice. With their heads full of questions and concerns and their hearts full of hope and fear, they fill the meditative void with mental meanderings, internal conversations, and questions without answers. Instead of making a vital connection between mind and body, they lose touch with their bodies and become lost in their heads.

Here's a technique I suggest to help my clients ground themselves lest their bodies levitate into the ether when they close their eyes and meditate. Use this simple exercise now, to merge mind and body and take hold of the opportunity before you. And use it in the future, whenever you need to be reminded that a calm and empty mind, a balanced body, and a willing set of hands are powerful tools for change.

While sitting comfortably, place your hands on your navel. Drop your jaw. Breathe deeply and slowly, letting each inhalation fill your abdomen; with each exhalation squeeze your PC (pubococcygeal) muscle gently. (To locate you PC muscle, see page 74.) Observe how your abdominal area rises and sinks with each breath. Now bring your awareness to your hands. Notice how they feel: Warm or cool? Calm or pulsing with energy? Before you open your eyes, imagine your hands becoming a more comfortable temperature, more energized, more aware—tools for carrying out the intent of your heart and mind.

to stick together and keep growing.) However, if you find you are not pregnant, you will want to avoid poultry during the first half of your cycle, when we want an open, not a constricted, environment in your body.

CHAPTER 4

FEED THE SEED: EATING AND DRINKING WISDOM

Early in this book, I asked you to empty your cup—to let go of preconceived notions and be open to a whole new way of thinking. Now it's
time to empty your *plate*—and take a whole new approach to the way you
nourish your body.

Before you read on, take note: The *Eating and Drinking Wisdom* you are
about to experience bears no resemblance to traditional Western food pyra-
mids or the advice you're likely to get from a Western nutritionist (or, for that
matter, a Western grandmother). In fact, these guidelines may seem to defy
Western logic, and often are not even emphasized by practitioners of Traditional Chinese Medicine because they puzzle Western eaters. They are, however, the very foundation of Traditional Chinese Medicine, which makes
little distinction among foods, beverages, and any medicine or herbs we
might put in our bodies; they are all part of the Five Elements continuum.

Traditional Chinese Medicine thinks about food and drink in a completely different way than Western medicine does. Instead of defining foods
according to their nutritional content—for example, how much vitamin B
or C they contain—Traditional Chinese Medicine looks at a food's *energetic*
nature: its impact on our vital fertility essences—remember Blood and
Qi?—and our internal weather.

Some foods are energetically *cool* or *cold,* regardless of their temperature.
When we eat them, they cool our bodies and affect our vital essences, other
foods are energetically *warm* or *hot,* regardless of their temperature. When
we eat them, they warm our bodies.

In addition, foods may be *constricting*, meaning they cause our essences and organs to contract, or *dispersing*, causing essences and organs to expand. They may also have *descending* energy, meaning they send Blood and Qi downward in our bodies, or *ascending* energy, sending Blood and Qi upwards.

Finally, some foods affect our internal weather by creating dampness. That dampness can either be cool, like a leaky basement, or warm, like a tropical forest. Dampness in the body most frequently manifests as mucus—something that we usually associate with the respiratory system, but that can also plague our digestive systems when we consistently eat foods that create dampness. But, in moderation, dampness can have a positive influence: For example, healthy sweets, including organic honey and dates, can slow down the body's energy, having a calming and stabilizing effect.

By understanding the energetic nature of the food we eat—whether it will warm or cool our bodies; cause Qi or Blood to expand, contract, ascend or descend; or create mucus—we can address whatever internal disharmony stands between our bodies and our babies by changing the way we nourish our bodies. (Remember: Tiny seeds need stable, harmonious, balanced weather to take root and thrive—neither too warm nor too cool, neither too dry nor too damp.) As we've already discussed, this *Eating and Drinking Wisdom* is a particularly powerful tool for women, whose fertility challenges tend to reside in the Blood—the vital essence we feed every time we eat and drink.

If, in chapter 2, you discovered that your internal weather tends to be cooler, you can bring your body into balance by adjusting your consumption patterns to eliminate energetically cold foods and emphasize more warming foods and beverages and cooking methods. If you discovered that your body usually runs warm, you can balance your internal weather by eliminating energetically hot foods, which cause or contribute to internal heat, and by introducing more foods that cool or clear heat. If you believe you have a

*You can alter the energetic properties of a food by the way you prepare or serve it. For example, by serving a warm-energy food at a cooler temperature, we can diminish its warming effect. And some cooking methods, such as roasting, add heat; others, like steaming, are cooler. To learn more, see "Fertility-Friendly Food Preparation Methods" on page 88.

combination constitution or you aren't sure which weather pattern fits you best, choose a variety of foods and beverages ranging from cool to neutral to warm to create a balanced and hospitable environment in your body.

With every meal, you have a new opportunity to balance Yin and Yang, harmonize the Five Elements, align your food and drink intake with your goal of conception, and create the ideal weather for new life. Bon appétit!

SOME FOOD FOR THOUGHT

Certain foods are hard on any body, whether its constitution is warmer or cooler. The foods described below—call it your *Don't!* list—are mainstays of many Westerners' diets and the source of many of the disharmonies I encounter in my practice. The better you can become at avoiding these foods, the better for your body, and your baby.

Processed, bleached foods: Think about the words "processed" and "bleached." They tell us right away that something has been altered in or removed from the foods they describe. From an Eastern perspective, eating these foods—particularly those made with white flour—is like covering up the sun; it keeps life-giving warmth away from the body. Energetically, wheat of any kind—even whole wheat—is cold, constricting, descending, and creates dampness, or mucus, in the body. It makes our Qi flow sluggishly and slows our digestive and metabolic processes, causing our bodies to store food as fat, not burn it as energy. If you simply cannot survive without flour-based foods, at least choose your grains carefully. A little sleuthing at your grocery or health food store may uncover breads, pastas, and even tortillas made with non-wheat flours, such as spelt or rice, that are better for your body.

Cold foods and drinks: Can you hear the voice of your Chinese grandmother? She's reminding you that chilled foods and drinks chill your body, causing your body temperature to drop and your circulation to slow. To boost circulation and maintain optimal body temperature, your heart must work harder—consuming the vital energy that you need for conception. So, for general good health—and particularly if you are trying to conceive or are already pregnant—*do not consume any foods or beverages cooler than room* *temperature.* That means nothing frozen (especially ice cream), nothing right out of the refrigerator, nothing with ice in it, and no water right from the "cold" tap. Whatever it is, heat it up or let it sit outside the fridge for an hour or so until it comes to room temperature (better yet, body temperature)—but please don't consume it cold.

Refined sweet foods: Energetically, sweetened and refined foods are both cold and damp—a double whammy of bad weather. Too much sweetness can overwhelm and weaken the spleen, slow digestion, and depress the immune system. (Did you know that eating or drinking just 100 grams of sugar—the amount in a can of soda—reduces your white blood cells' ability to fight germs by 40 percent?) So for the sake of your baby, forgo cakes, cookies, candies, and other snacks laden with sucrose, dextrose, corn syrup, brown sugar, turbinado sugar, or molasses, and choose fruit (which is also sweet but may benefit your body—see "A Word about Fruit" on page 81) with care. Honey is the most fertility-friendly sweetener. But please be sure it's natural or organic, with no sugar added, and practice moderation.

Dairy products: Most dairy products (such as milk, cheese, and butter) create dampness—mucus—that hampers the flow of Qi through the body's energy meridians. Over time, impeding the flow of any essence—Blood or Qi—can create stagnation which is not an ideal condition for conception and pregnancy. The only dairy product I recommend to my fertility clients is low-fat cottage cheese. In its drier, curd form (and eaten in moderation), it does not generate the overwhelming dampness of other dairy foods, so it is a safe source of calcium.

Old food: No one likes to see good leftovers go to waste. And many of us, for convenience in our busy lives, like to cook in large quantities and feast on the same foods during the course of the week. But did you know that, after less than 24 hours, the nutritional value and Qi in cooked foods begin to deteriorate rapidly, even in the refrigerator? In Traditional Chinese Medicine, we regard cooked foods that have sat around for more than 24 hours as "dead"—diminished in nutritional value, more difficult to digest, and contributing to dampness in our bodies. When you're eating in preparation for pregnancy, you need maximum nutritional value from the foods you consume. Therefore, make sure the foods you put in your body are freshly cooked (or, if uncooked, are fresh) and alive with Qi—no matter how good and easy that casserole may sound on Day 3.

A note about deep freezes: Even when thawed properly and prepared promptly, foods that have been frozen don't have the same Qi as fresh foods. However, if they have sustained the cold well (meaning no freezer burn) and have not been in your freezer since the Ice Age, they can be acceptable and convenient additions to a meal that also includes fresh foods.

Extreme Energy Foods: Foods that have extremely hot or extremely cold energy can have a profound impact on your body, but not necessarily in the way you might expect. Extreme energy foods are an interesting example of the fifth principal of Yin and Yang at work, in which Yin and Yang become each other. They can catalyze what we call "disharmonious transformation," in which, for example, a food is so hot it actually chills your body, or so cold it creates heat. Again, because we are striving for balance and harmony, we want to avoid extremes of all kinds, particularly when those extremes can transform our internal temperature in disharmonious ways.

One final thought: Some foods are especially hard on the body because

 A WORD ABOUT FRUIT

Although many fruits, with their natural sugars, are sweet, our *Eating and Drinking Wisdom* makes room for fruit if you choose carefully. (In fact, some people find that the natural sugars in fruit have a calming effect for them—in contrast to the dramatic energy highs and lows we experience when we eat artificially sweetened foods.) In my practice, unless a client's internal weather is very cool and could be compromised by any raw food, I may encourage the occasional apple, asian pear, raspberries, or red or purple grapes. (An apple baked with a little honey is a tasty and fertility-friendly treat, popular with many of my clients.) And although it's energetically a cold fruit, a banana first thing in the morning, followed by a glass of warm water, is a good remedy for chronic constipation (a sign of heat), as well as a good source of potassium. However, I advise all clients to avoid pineapple, mango, and other energetically hot fruits, as well as melons and other fruits that have cold energy. And I recommend against eating fruit in colder weather, or during the winter season, when your body needs more warming, cooked foods.

they combine several energetic negatives. For example, ice cream is frozen, it's a refined sweet, and it's a dairy product—a surefire way to create Qi-sapping cold and dampness in your body. The same goes for pizza: It combines energetically damp wheat, sweet tomato sauce, and mucus-causing cheese. If you're a pizza and ice cream fan—and you're serious about overcoming your body's challenges to pregnancy—my advice is that you cultivate new, energetically healthier food preferences. A slice of pizza and a hot fudge sundae may taste good on your tongue, but in your body, they are a recipe for stormy weather.

Charlie and Will's Story
(DON'T) LET THEM EAT CAKE

*D*octors told Marcia that there was no medical reason she couldn't conceive. So, after 13 years of trying, where was her baby?

When she and her husband, Bill, came to our clinic, it was Marcia's tongue that revealed the keenest insight into the probable source of their problems. Its pallor betrayed the cool, damp constitution I often see in women with a sweet tooth.

Together Marcia and Bill decided that they would work hard to bring Marcia's body into balance and harmony by strictly following the Fertility Wisdom *program for 3 to 6 months before expecting to conceive. For Marcia that meant replacing sweets, wheat, and dairy products with cooked meats and vegetables conducive to creating a warm, baby-friendly internal environment. It was a challenging shift but, Marcia and Bill believed, worth the effort.*

Everything went well until the 3rd month: It was Marcia's birthday and, frustrated after months of the "deprivation diet," she wanted cake. Bill gently reminded her of their priorities: Wasn't all the progress they'd made—and the hope of the baby they'd wanted for 13 years—worth more than cake? With Bill's help, Marcia overcame her craving, and by the end of the 3rd month, she was pregnant with Charlie.

A year or so later, Marcia and Bill decided to expand their family. With help from Western fertility treatments, Marcia conceived, only to miscarry early in her pregnancy. Afterward, Marcia and Bill re-embraced the Eastern concepts that had enabled Marcia to conceive and carry Charlie full term, and Will was born. When the family visited San Francisco so that its youngest members could see their own faces on our wall of acubaby photos, I wished them all life's sweetest gifts (but I did not serve their mother cake).

EATING FOR THE WEATHER— INSIDE AND OUT

In the Taoist view of things, our bodies are part of the greater environment they inhabit, governed by the same laws and affected by the same seasonal changes in energy. As you feed your internal garden in preparation for pregnancy, there are four climatic influences we will be taking into consideration.

Internal weather: By this, I am referring to your constitutional pattern—warmer or cooler. If you have determined that you have a cooler constitution, you'll want to take care to avoid cold or cool foods and make sure you're eating enough warm foods. If you have a warmer constitution, you'll want to avoid foods that add heat (hot and warm foods) and find ways to add gently cooling foods to your meals. If you don't feel comfortable defining yourself as either warmer or cooler, you can choose foods and beverages that reinforce well-balanced internal weather. Your rule of thumb: Avoid foods on the hot and cold ends of the spectrum, and choose a balanced variety of foods that are warm, cool, or neutral.

Outdoor weather/season of the year: What's it like outside? Is it a warm July day or a cold January night? As the seasons shift and the weather changes day to day, our food and beverage intake can shift as well—more warming foods to compensate for the energy our bodies lose to the environment on cold days; more cooling foods to help our bodies stay healthy and hydrated on hot days. Equally important, we can take special care to avoid cold foods on cold days and to avoid hot foods when the weather outside is already adding heat to our internal landscape. And as the seasons and weather shift, we can adapt our eating and drinking habits—for example, eating a bit more fruit or a little salad as the weather warms up. (One piece of advice: If you change your food and beverage intake, add no more than one new item at a time, and consume it in moderation; that way, you can test its impact on your internal weather.)

Immediate environment: Where do you spend most of your day? In an air-conditioned office or over a hot stove? If you consistently spend time in a cool environment, don't be surprised if your internal weather is also cool. If you spend most of your time in a warm place, you may find that your body also shows signs of heat. You can balance the impact of your immediate environment through food and drink—for example, making sure you drink enough water if you work in a warm environment. But don't forget: You can also choose to change your environment to one that is more conducive to conception and pregnancy.

BALANCING BODY AND ENVIRONMENT

To eat in sync with the season or the day's weather, follow these simple guidelines:

When it's hot and/or dry outside . . .

- Take special care to avoid energetically hot foods and drinks.
- Avoid cooking methods that add warmth to food (e.g., deep-frying).
- Make sure you drink water—at room temperature or body temperature—when you're becoming thirsty.
- If you have a warmer constitution, look for opportunities to eat a few cooling foods or serve warmer-energy foods at a cooler temperature.

When it's chilly outside . . .

- Take special care to avoid energetically cold foods and drinks, as well as chilled or iced drinks and foods cooler than room temperature.
- If you have a cooler constitution, look for opportunities to eat a few warming foods or foods cooked using a method that adds a little warmth (e.g., baking, roasting) or serve cooler-energy foods at a warmer temperature.

Activity level: How active you are has an impact on your body's weather. Vigorous physical activity adds warmth; gentle exercise and rest have a cooling effect. So if your constitution, the weather outside, or your immediate environment is cooler, you can warm things up with physical activity. Likewise, you can balance warmer influences with rest and gentle activity, such as stretches or the Six Healing Sounds, a Taoist practice you'll learn more about in chapter 6.

A WORD ABOUT RAW

In an era when many Westerners regard raw food as the ultimate source of uncompromised nutrition, avoiding raw foods may seem outrageous. But for many women, it couldn't be more critical to creating the ideal environment for conception. Time and again in my clinic, I see women with cooler constitutions who seem to subsist on salads, fruit, and juice because they think raw food is more nutritious. Little do they know that their bodies are spending so much Qi digesting raw foods that they have little left to support conception and pregnancy.

Simply put, raw foods require more energy to digest than cooked foods. Cooking helps break down food structure, making it easier for our bodies to use essential nutrients. Cooking also warms food, and eating warm food warms our bodies—particularly important for people with cooler constitutions, when the weather is cold, or when it's winter. And when food is close to our *body temperature*—that is, warm—we need less energy to digest it.

So the next time you're considering a salad or even a carrot stick, stop for a moment and ask yourself: Is this the best source of nutrition for my body right now? Remember: Eating raw food can take more than it gives back. If your body doesn't have enough Qi to process them, raw-food nutrients end up being excreted.

Before incorporating raw foods in your diet, consider the following guidelines.

Internal weather: If you have a cooler constitution, do your Qi a favor and eat food that is cooked and warm instead of food that is raw and cool. If your constitution is warmer, a little raw food—at the right time of day, the right time of year, and in the right weather (read on to learn more) won't hurt. And if you have signs of stagnation as well as a warmer constitution, a modest amount of raw food can be beneficial. (For example, it's very important that women who have uterine fibroids, a classic sign of Blood stagnation, maintain a diet that generates a healthy bowel movement, which will carry toxins out of the body. Eating plenty of fresh vegetables—including salad greens—is a good way to achieve this goal.)

Time of day: Because we are eating to balance Yin and Yang in our bodies as well as to harmonize the Five Elements, there are some times of day that are better for raw foods than others. As a general guideline, if you choose

---

 WISDOM FOR EVERY WEATHER

When nourishing your body with food and drink . . .

Avoid

- Wheat
- Refined sweets
- Dairy
- Processed or bleached foods
- Coffee and soft drinks
- Alcohol
- Iced, chilled, or frozen foods or drinks
- Extreme foods and drinks (those foods listed as energetically hot or cold in the Food Energies chart on page 89) and preparation methods (e.g., deep-frying)

Favor

- Foods listed in the neutral energetic category in the "Food Energies" table on page 89
- Body or room temperature or warm beverages
- Freshly cooked foods
- A wide variety of foods compatible with your internal weather
- A wide variety of flavors, reflecting all the Five Elements: sweet, sour, salty, bitter, pungent

to eat raw foods, which are more Yin, it's best to consume them at more Yang times of day—for example, at lunch. In general, be sure that the first foods you put in your body in the morning are cooked, and avoid raw foods after sundown.

Time of year: Yin and Yang play out across the seasons much as they do throughout the day, and we eat best when we eat in harmony with these patterns. In winter, when days are shorter and the weather tends to be cooler, choose cooked foods that warm your body over raw foods that take precious Qi to digest. In summer, when Yang energy is at its peak and the Fire element dominates, our bodies are better able to process raw foods.

Outside weather: Even in summer, there can be cool, rainy days, just as in winter we may get an unexpected burst of heat. When the weather is warm, our bodies are better able to digest raw foods; when it's cool and damp, choose something cooked.

Activity level: Since your body needs energy to digest raw food, it's best to avoid raw if you're tired or engaging in activities that deplete your energy. (Tired after a busy day on the run? Choose cooked foods that will restore your energy.) On the other hand, if you're engaging in activity that revitalizes you, you'll have more of the energy you need to digest raw food. (Invigorated after a gentle stroll? A little raw is okay.) Learn to listen to your body.

REMEMBER . . .

If your internal weather is warm:

- Avoid energetically hot foods.
- Drink when you're thirsty.
- Favor "juicy" foods that provide the fluids your body needs.
- Avoid cooking methods that add warmth to food (such as roasting or deep-frying); favor methods that minimize heat (such as steaming).

If your internal weather is cool:

- Avoid energetically cold foods.
- Eat foods and drink beverages at room temperature or warmer.
- Favor denser foods (such as root vegetables) that generate more warmth when digested.
- Favor cooking methods that add warmth to food (such as roasting or sautéing).

If you have stagnation:

- Avoid heavy foods.

FILLING YOUR PLATE

The charts that follow tell you the energetic nature, from hot to cold, of a variety of foods and beverages—some familiar, some strange and new. Some of these associations will make sense intuitively. (For example, you may have already noticed that garlic, scallions, gingerroot, and pepper warm up the body.) Others may surprise you. (Would you have guessed that peaches are one of the "hottest" fruits, or that pork has a cooling energy?)

Before you explore these lists, I urge you, once again, to "empty your cup" of preconceptions and prepare for a whole new way of relating to the nourishment you put in your body. Instead of counting calories or assessing nutrient content, you will be striving for balance and harmony—a diet that is neither too warm nor too cool and that samples the amazing variety of foods, beverages, herbs, and spices nature provides.

Putting together a nutritious, satisfying meal plan that also balances and harmonizes your internal weather may sound like a tall task, but it can be done, with perseverance, a sense of adventure, and a little imagination. For inspiration, consult Appendix D on page 211, where you'll find tips and sample menus for cultivating a receptive, baby-friendly internal environment.

 FERTILITY-FRIENDLY FOOD PREPARATION METHODS

The way a food is prepared has an impact on its energetic quality. Our *Eating and Drinking Wisdom* prefers preparation methods that allow us to access the nutrition in food without adding too much heat or bringing too cool an influence to our bodies—for example, steaming, boiling, stewing, stir-frying, or sautéing. (In general, longer cooking adds more warmth to a food.) However, you can also render a hot food more fertility friendly by using a cooler method to prepare it, or you can warm a cool-energy food by using a warmer cooking technique.

Cooling: Raw

Neutral: Steamed, boiled

Warming: Stewed, stir-fried, sautéed

Heating: Baked

Hottest: Deep-fried, roasted, grilled, barbecued

FOOD ENERGIES

In Traditional Chinese Medicine, we assess a food's value by its energy rather than by its nutritional content as measured in calories, vitamins, or minerals. As you eat to balance your body in preparation for a baby, this chart will be your guide to the energies of common foods. The best baby weather is neither hot nor cold. Depending on your constitution (warm? cool? stagnant?), you'll be choosing foods in the cool-to-warm range. When in doubt, eat "neutral."

COLD	COOL	NEUTRAL	WARM	HOT
VEGETABLES				
Celery	Alfalfa	Chard	Bell pepper	Carrot
Chinese cabbage	Asparagus	Green and	Chinese chive	Garlic
Cucumber	Bamboo shoot	red cabbage	Chinese leafy	Ginger
Mung bean	Beet	Pea	broccoli	Scallion
sprout	Bok choy	Shiitake mush-	Ganoderma	
Mustard greens	Broccoli	room	mushroom	
Seaweed	Burdock root	Sweet potato	Green or red	
Snow pea	Button mush-	Taro root	cabbage	
Water chestnut	room	Yam	Green string	
White mush-	Cauliflower		bean	
room	Corn		Leek	
	Daikon radish		Onion	
	Dandelion		Parsley	
	greens		Parsnip	
	Eggplant		Pumpkin	
	Endive			
	Kale			
	Lettuce			
	Lotus root			
	Napa cabbage			
	Potato			
	Romaine lettuce			
	Spinach			
	Sprouts			
	Summer squash			
	Turnip			
	Watercress			
	Winter melon			
	Winter squash			
	Zucchini			

continued on page 90

FOOD ENERGIES				
COLD	**COOL**	**NEUTRAL**	**WARM**	**HOT**
FRUITS				
Banana	Blueberry	Apple	Cherry	Apricot
Cantaloupe	Lemon	Chinese date	Chinese	Nectarine
Grapefruit	Pear	Coconut	plum	Peach
Honeydew mel-	Pear-apple	Loquat	Fig	Purple grapes
on	Persimmon	Olive	Grape	
Mulberry	Strawberry	Papaya (fresh)	Hawthorn	
Watermelon	Tomato	Plum	berry	
		Yellow grapes	Lychee	
			Mango	
			Orange	
			Papaya	
			(dried)	
			Pineapple	
			Raspberry	
			Red	
			grapes	
			Tangerine	
GRAINS				
Barley	Brown rice	Buckwheat	Oat	Millet
	Fresh bread	Cornmeal	Sweet rice	
	Pearl barley	Rice bran	Wheat bran	
	Wheat	Rye	Wheat germ	
		White rice		
NUTS, SEEDS, AND BEANS				
Mung bean	Black bean	Almond	Brown sesame	Black sesame
Pumpkin seed	Kidney bean	Azuki bean	seed	seed
	Miso	Filbert	Chestnut	
	Tofu	Lotus seed	Lentil	
	Winter melon	Peanut	Pine nut	
	seed	Soybean	Red bean	
		Sunflower	Walnut	
		seed		

FOOD ENERGIES				
COLD	**COOL**	**NEUTRAL**	**WARM**	**HOT**
ANIMAL PRODUCTS				
Mussel Pork Yogurt	Clam Cottage cheese Crab Fish (ocean) Milk Oyster Shrimp	All eggs Fish (fresh- water) Gelatin Herring Most dairy products Black-bone chicken	Beef Chicken Turkey	Eel Lamb Venison
MEDICINAL AND CULINARY HERBS AND SPICES				
Bamboo shav- ing Cassia seed Chinese cucum- ber Chrysanthe- mum Goldenseal root Honeysuckle flower Motherwort leaf Mulberry leaf Oyster shell Reed root	American gin- seng Cilantro Corn silk Kudzu (puer- aria) Lily flower Mint leaf Mint tea Pueraria root	Chinese yam Licorice root Lycii berry Poria mush- room	Anise seed Asian ginseng Basil Cardamom seed Carob pod Citrus peel Clove Coriander seed Dang gui Fennel seed Fresh ginger	Black pepper Cinnamon bark Dry ginger Garlic Korean red gin- seng
MISCELLANEOUS				
Salt Salty, sour, and sweet pickle and relish Vitamin C White sugar	Chamomile tea Green tea Mint tea	Barley malt Black fungus Honey Rice malt White fungus	Black tea Brown sugar Coffee Molasses Raspberry leaf tea Vinegar Wine	Spicy pickle and relish

IF YOU ARE WHAT YOU EAT, WHO ARE YOU?

Before making any changes in what you eat and drink, let's explore how what you already consume might be influencing your internal weather. For the next week, keep track of everything you eat as well as its temperature (for example, right out of the refrigerator, room temperature, or heated). Write down everything, even things you know you shouldn't be eating or drinking! (An honest assessment is your most powerful tool for improvement.)

At the end of the week, review your eating and drinking diary against the Food Energies chart on pages 89-91. Jot down the energetic value—cold, cool, neutral, warm, or hot—of each item (or of its main ingredients, if it's a dish composed of many things). When you glance at the energies of the items you consumed over the last week, what patterns emerge? Do you notice a preponderance of foods or drinks at either extreme of the hot to cold spectrum? Do you seem to be consuming a lot of raw foods? Refrigerated foods or beverages? Does your diet lean heavily on wheat and dairy products? Is it balanced and varied, or does it concentrate on just a few foods?

Now take a minute to size up your food and drink intake against what you know about your internal weather. If your constitution is warmer, what foods might be adding heat to your system? If your constitution is cooler, what items might be contributing to your chilly condition? As you proceed with this program, look for opportunities to replace foods and drinks that reinforce disharmonious internal weather with new foods and drinks that balance and harmonize your body.

Bobby's Story
GIVING UP A BIRTHDAY FOR A BIRTH

*K*elly had worked hard to stay healthy. She biked and swam and stayed toned through yoga. She stuck to what most people consider a faultlessly healthy diet: lots of raw fruits and vegetables, very little meat. But within a little more than a year, Kelly had *miscarried three times—always between week 8 and week 11 of pregnancy.*

Sad and discouraged, Kelly consulted a fertility expert, whose diagnosis did nothing to improve her spirits: At 39, her eggs were just too old, said the expert. Her best bet for a baby would be through Assisted Reproductive Technology (ART). So Kelly consented to Western fertility treatments and took two courses of Clomid, a drug commonly used to induce ovulation. Nothing happened.

When Kelly visited our clinic, I saw in her tongue and pulses the signs of a cooler constitution exacerbated by too much raw food. Trained as a nurse, Kelly was skeptical, but she agreed to embrace the strange new Eating and Drinking Wisdom, *even though it turned her long-held beliefs about nutrition upside down.*

Within just a few weeks, Kelly was pregnant—naturally. Her question was, could she stay pregnant? My answer: Not unless she parked her bike, stayed out of the pool, and temporarily gave up yoga—beloved activities that threatened the viability of the delicate seed she was carrying. The compromise made her sad, but for the sake of her baby, Kelly persevered—until the day she announced to me that she would be flying to Europe to celebrate her father's 70th birthday. Aware of the fragility of her condition, I advised against it, and Kelly protested. After all, her father would only turn 70 once. "You're right," I said. "Let your gift to him be the healthy baby that results when you stay home through your first trimester."

It wasn't easy to miss a landmark in her family's history, but as families will, her father and other relatives understood. A few months later, when they welcomed Bobby, everyone agreed that missing a birthday was a fair trade for a healthy birth. And when Kelly's best friend, Sarah, who'd also suffered a miscarriage, conceived with help from our Fertility Wisdom *program and delivered her baby not long afterward, Kelly's happiness doubled.*

WHAT IF YOU'RE A VEGETARIAN?

Although a modest amount of the right meats offers benefits to women seeking to boost fertility (protein and a source of warmth), vegetarians also can use our *Eating and Drinking Wisdom* to improve their chances of conceiving. Check the Food Energies chart on pages 89-91 for protein alternatives—beans, nuts, avocado—that complement your internal weather. For example, you can tell a bean's energetic nature by its color: Green beans such as mung (representing Wood and Spring among the Five Elements) are cooler, so they're better for warmer constitutions; red beans (Fire and Summer) are warmer, making them good for cooler internal weather; and soybeans (Earth and Indian Summer) are neutral.

COMBINING FOODS FOR GREATER NUTRITION

In addition to choosing foods based on your constitution, you can optimize your body's energy by combining foods in ways that make them easy to digest.

Here's how it works: Different foods require different digestive environments to break them down effectively. For example, starches digest best when your stomach is more alkaline, proteins when it is more acidic. But alkaline and acid neutralize each other, so if you put a protein and most forms of starch (for example, potatoes or pasta) in your stomach at the same time, you create a neutral gastric environment that digests neither food properly. Undigested food ferments in your digestive tract, eventually leading to problems, from gas to constipation.

If you eat more than one food at a meal (as most of us do), you can greatly improve your digestion by combining foods that require the same gastric juices. Here are a few simple guidelines for you to try:

- Eat starches and proteins at separate meals. (One exception: White rice can be eaten with meat, particularly in an easily digestible soup.)
- Eat only one kind of protein per meal. (For example, eat nuts and cheese at separate meals.)

- Eat high-fat foods and proteins at separate meals.
- Combine green leafy vegetables with proteins or starches—but not with both.
- Skip desserts. Eaten after a heavy meal, they tend to ferment in the stomach.
- Remember that digestion begins in your mouth. Chew all foods thoroughly.

You can also improve your digestion by eating foods in a particular order. Cooked, warming foods (including meats) should be consumed at the beginning of the meal. If you're eating cooler foods, these should be consumed at the end of the meal. Why? Because, when we eat, we want to mimic the rhythms of the seasons: Warming our bodies at the beginning of the meal (Spring) and eating cooler foods later in the meal as our bodies warm up (Summer).

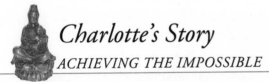

Charlotte's Story
ACHIEVING THE IMPOSSIBLE

"*You've got to be kidding!*" *That's what Naomi said to me when I explained the new way she would have to eat and drink in order to bring her body into fertility-ready harmony.*

Interestingly, those words echo the prognosis given Naomi when she first started trying to conceive naturally. She'd wanted to have a child as long as she could remember, and as time passed, she wondered if she would ever find a life partner and raise a family. Then she met Terry, and the first part of the puzzle fell into place. She was 39 at the time, and her doctors gave her one directive: Get pregnant before your 40th birthday if you really want to have a baby, because the clock is ticking.

When she and Terry had difficulty conceiving, Naomi attributed

AND THERE'S MORE!

In addition to the *Eating and Drinking Wisdom* I've shared on these pages, I also recommend the following supplements to help ensure that women and men obtain the essential vitamins and minerals they need every day.

For women

- 1,600 milligrams of folic acid per day
- Prenatal vitamins and other supplements as recommended by your doctor or nutritionist (be sure to count the folic acid in your prenatal vitamin toward your total daily intake)

For men

- Selenium
- Antioxidants (available in green tea and many vegetables—especially green vegetables)
- B Vitamin complex
- Zinc

the trouble to surgeries she'd had in her twenties: She'd had one ovary removed and had a cyst taken from the other ovary. Tests also showed that Terry had a low sperm count. With the possibility of a natural pregnancy looking slim, doctors recommended intrauterine insemination or in vitro fertilization as their best options.

But Naomi and Terry wanted an alternative, and they found one in Traditional Chinese Medicine. Immediately I recommended that Naomi, with her cooler constitution, eliminate cold foods and beverages and use warming foods to balance her body. At first, Naomi feared the cure would prove worse than the ailment: Giving up ice cream, wheat, and other beloved foods would be impossible, particularly on their belated honeymoon in Paris. But the two persevered; Terry even tried our seemingly unorthodox food approach— including a special Chinese soup of black-boned chicken and seahorse (yes, seahorse—the only species whose males carry and deliver the babies), a traditional Eastern fertility remedy for men. After 3 months of balancing and harmonizing, Naomi conceived naturally—the weekend before her 40th birthday.

Convinced of the impact of Traditional Chinese Medicine, Naomi stuck to the program (including the dreaded eating and drinking guidelines) to prevent a first-trimester miscarriage. In due time Charlotte was born, demonstrating that birthday wishes can come true.

A SPECIAL NOTE ON WATER

You've heard it your whole life: Drink eight glasses of water a day. And although it's true that you must provide your body with enough fresh water every day to moisten your tissues and organs and keep all systems operating properly, this is one situation where we will refine Grandmother's advice: We all need enough water, but not all of us need eight glasses. Some of us need more. Some of us need less.

How can you tell how much water you need? In China, there's a saying: Don't eat when you're hungry; eat before you're hungry. The same can be said for thirst: Drink *before* you become thirsty or notice signs of dehydration, such as dry mouth, nostrils, and/or eyes; dark yellow urine; or hard, dry bowel movements.

A general tip: Because they burn through fluids quickly, warmer constitutions tend to need more water to keep the body from becoming dehydrated. Those with cooler constitutions may need less water and should be certain that whatever water they drink is no colder than room temperature—warm water is even better. The ideal water temperature for all constitutions is body temperature.

Anything we put in our stomachs affects our body temperature and the digestion of whatever foods are already in the digestive tract. For example, you don't want to throw cold water on your stomach while it's digesting a heavy meal; you'll dilute critical gastric juices and compromise your body's ability to render food into nutrition.

So, ideally, drink water that is at body temperature, and at intervals that don't affect your body's ability to digest food. For example, 15 minutes

EATING AND DRINKING TIPS

- Plan a full day's meals in advance so that you can balance what you eat across all meals.
- Attending a dinner party or family function? Don't go hungry—bring rice cakes, rye crackers (made without wheat or flour), hummus, low-fat cottage cheese, or another fertility-friendly snack so you know you will have enough to eat.
- Attending a barbecue? Bring rice-based bread so you can enjoy a burger.
- Eating out? Get in the habit of asking for "water without ice." (In fact, if you drink water well before you go out, your undiluted gastric juices will process your meal more effectively.) Substitute a soup for a salad as your starter. And don't be afraid to ask for substitutions—for example, rice pilaf instead of pasta or potato.
- Learn to read labels carefully. Be on the lookout for hidden sugars (including high-fructose corn syrup) and refined flours, and avoid products that list these items close to the top of the ingredients list.
- Cooking for multiple eaters? Prepare "mix-and-match" meals that let diners prepare the plate of their choice—for example, they enjoy the pasta side dish with their meal, you enjoy the main course and green vegetable.
- Expand your shopping territory. If you're used to shopping at the same corner store or local mega-market, make an effort to investigate new alternatives—for example, farmers' markets, organic grocers, health food stores, or Asian markets, if you have any in your community (they are good sources of rice-based noodles). You might also check to see if your local grocery store has an Asian foods, health foods, or wheat-free section.
- Avoid fruit and vegetable juices. Because they contain the "essence" of many individual items (for example, three carrots in a single glass of juice), they tend to create dampness. If you do drink them, dilute them with water.
- Investigate online sources. Many of our clients have found wheat substitutes and other fertility-friendly food alternatives by shopping the Internet.
- Use your imagination—and listen to your body. If you're expanding your eating repertoire, try to add only one new food at a time. Then pay attention to how you feel the day after eating it.

before any meal is a good time to drink water. Avoid drinking during a meal (though a sip or two of water is okay). Wait 15 minutes after a vegetarian meal, 30 minutes after a starchy meal, and 1 hour after a protein meal before drinking larger quantities of water.

STOCKING A FERTILITY-FRIENDLY PANTRY

You'll be more likely to stick to our *Eating and Drinking Wisdom* if your pantry is full of healthy options. Before embarking on the *Fertility Wisdom* program, take a shopping trip and stock up on a few fertility-friendly staples.

- Olive oil: For sautéing and dressing foods.
- Flax seed oil: A wonderful source of antioxidants, but it must be refrigerated and should not be heated. Use to dress vegetables.
- Sesame oil: A warming oil, so use in moderation (and only on occasion) to add flavor or gently warm a cooler constitution (or to make Ama's Post-Period/Postpartum Poached Chicken or Eggs, on page 71).
- Rice wine: Use to make Ama's Post-Period/Postpartum Poached Chicken or Eggs.
- Fresh ginger: Eaten raw or in its dried form, ginger disperses energy and should be avoided. But when cooked, it greatly aids digestion. Add a slice to rice while you're cooking it, or sauté with vegetables, such as greens.
- Garlic: Valuable for its antibiotic properties; consume cooked only.
- Scallions: Two foods in one: Cook the white part of the bulb gently to add warmth to a dish; add chopped scallion tops toward the end of cooking.
- Oats: Rolled or steel cut; a good breakfast option.
- Dried apple slices and raisins: Turn to these when you want something sweet, but please use moderation. (You may also steam a fresh apple— if you promise to eat apples in moderation!)

- Honey: The safest of the sweets; use in moderation.
- Raw nuts: Walnuts, almonds, cashews; no more than a handful a day.
- Green tea: The safest and most beneficial form of caffeine; high in antioxidants, and with cooling properties that benefit a warmer constitution. Also a good beverage for detoxing after Western fertility treatments. Avoid if you have a cooler constitution with no signs of heat.
- Long-grain white rice: For example, basmati. White rice, steamed or in congee, is one starch that is good eaten with meats; it helps your body digest protein.
- Rice-based noodles: Available in a variety of shapes; check your local health food store or Asian market.
- Rice-based bread products: For example, breads and tortillas. You may also be able to find bread products that use spelt or kamut flour instead of wheat flour. Choose brands that do not include any wheat flour.
- Low-fat cottage cheese: Of all dairy products, the least likely to cause internal dampness; a good source of calcium.
- Rice cakes: A good alternative to breads and a healthy, easy-to-transport snack.
- Rice milk: For drinking or use with non-wheat cereals.
- Vegetable broth: Many health food stores carry vegetable powder that can be made into a broth; you may also find vegetable broths in cartons (which should be refrigerated after opening).
- Wheat-free tamari: A fertility-friendly alternative to soy sauce. Use in moderation as a marinade or dressing.
- Sea salt: An easy-to-digest seasoning.
- Ground black pepper: A little is good for the pre-ovulation phase, when women need to maintain a warm constitution; avoid it post ovulation, when it can disperse energy, or if you have a warmer constitution.
- Canned or dried beans: Particularly important for vegetarians as a source of protein, as well as a source of fiber. Consult the Food Energies charts on pages 89-91 for options that suit your particular constitution.

- Grain alternatives: For example, quinoa, an increasingly popular and available grain, is a good source of protein. Much like rice, it can be steamed or made into a pilaf using vegetable stock or water.
- Meats to suit your constitution (organic if possible): A little beef for most constitutions, a little lamb to warm a cooler constitution (particularly in winter), a little pork for warmer constitutions, and poultry for after ovulation. Black-bone cicken, a fertility-friendly poultry alternative for women and men, nourishes Qi and Blood. (See recipe on page 218.)
- Fish: Choose low-mercury options; prepare steamed or sautéed; avoid shellfish.
- Plenty of fresh (organic) vegetables: Consult the Food Energies chart on page 89 for a variety of options, avoiding vegetables in the Cold or Hot energetic categories.
- An easy source of fresh, healthy, room- or body-temperature water: Bottled or filtered and kept out of the refrigerator.

 I JUST CAN'T DO THIS!

If giving up foods like wheat, cold drinks, and ice cream just seems too difficult, try this: Listen to your body. How do you feel after eating these foods? Once you learn to tune in to your body, you may notice that an iced drink has an immediate impact: You feel colder! Also observe your body's reactions within a day or so of consuming something "forbidden." How is your energy the day after you've eaten pizza?

If you have an irregular menstrual cycle or your flow is too heavy or too light, try avoiding foods on the *Don't!* list for 1 month and see if your patterns change.

Finally, ask yourself: Is the short-term satisfaction of these foods worth missing out on parenthood? If you're only adhering to the eating and drinking guidelines 75 percent of the time, is 75 percent successful good enough for you? (To be honest, I've never seen anyone who was 75 percent pregnant.)

NOURISHING YOUR FUTURE

Warm, cool, constricting, dispersing, ascending, descending—feeling overwhelmed by a new food vocabulary that bears no resemblance to any menu you've ever seen? You are not alone.

Embracing our *Eating and Drinking Wisdom* has been a challenge for many of the people who've used this program. I see it every day at my clinic: stubborn resistance ("I can't live without chocolate!"), complaints ("It's impossible for me to give up wheat; it's in everything!" or "My husband thinks it's weird!"), cajoling ("Please, please—won't you let me have just one salad a day?"), bargaining ("If I give up iced tea, can I have ice cream?" or "What if I drink my white wine warm?"). Some claim the sense of deprivation they feel is increasing their stress levels—a convenient excuse for eating half a chocolate cake or a bag of cashews.

Over time, however, these protestations give way to happy surprise when, low and behold, once-irregular periods start to arrive like clockwork, FSH levels drop, sleep improves, energy goes up, mood swings diminish—and people just feel better and more hopeful.

Of course, some clients bend the eating and drinking guidelines to fit what they're able (or willing) to give up. (They may not confess to me, but I can always tell—their bodies don't lie.) I encourage them to stick as closely as possible to these guidelines for at least the first three to six months of the *Fertility Wisdom* program in order to bring their bodies into better balance and harmony. Then they can add new foods—one food at a time, and no more than one day per week—observing carefully to see how their bodies respond. Whether you adhere to these guidelines strictly or choose to compromise, there are some things I know for certain: Those who adopt our *Eating and Drinking Wisdom* have a greater chance of conceiving and carrying their babies full term. Those who embrace this new way of nourishing their bodies—through pregnancy, post-pregnancy, for the rest of their lives—are healthier and happier for it. And every single one of them will tell you: Their babies make them much happier than ice cream ever did.

CHAPTER 5

NURTURE YOUR ORGANS: ACUPRESSURE TECHNIQUES

Take a moment to give yourself credit for everything you've accomplished in your quest for pregnancy. You've begun to change unhealthy habits—smoking and drinking, not getting enough rest, exercising too much or too little—that may have been with you for years. You're adjusting the way you eat and drink to create a more harmonious and balanced internal environment. And you're taking extra precautions after ovulation—avoiding disruptions of all kinds; eating poultry to secure a possible pregnancy—to protect the potential new life inside you. In short, you've begun to nurture yourself.

Now it's time to focus that nurturing *inward*—on the organs whose health reflects harmonious internal weather.

In chapter 1, we talked about how your liver, heart, spleen, lungs, and kidneys relate to the Five Elements—Wood, Fire, Earth, Metal, and Water. To practitioners of Traditional Chinese Medicine, the health of these organs reflects the relationship among the Five Elements, and vice versa: When the Five Elements are out of harmony, our organs are, too.

How do our bodies fall into disharmony? In some cases, we may inherit a tendency toward disharmony through the prenatal Qi we receive from our parents. Sometimes we create our own disharmony through the ways we eat, drink, and care for our bodies. (For example, years of energetically cold, refrigerator-chilled, raw foods can greatly deplete a constitution so that it runs cooler.) And often it's the way we process (or fail to process) everyday stress that contributes to disharmony in our bodies.

Think about what happens to your body when you're upset, under pressure, or overworked. Your muscles tighten up. Maybe your stomach hurts. You might get headaches or suffer from constipation or diarrhea. These symptoms are the outermost manifestations of disturbances taking place much deeper in your body— at the organ level.

To relieve these symptoms and truly restore inner harmony, we can do more than take an aspirin or an antacid; these are temporary remedies to problems that will only recur the next time we're under stress. We can nurture our organs using practical techniques that are as old as Chinese medicine itself—and were once the privileged knowledge of Taoist sages devoted to cultivating healthy internal weather.

WISDOM DOWN FROM THE MOUNTAIN

At the end of the introduction, when you first set aside Western preconceptions by "emptying your cup," we left a young scholar atop a mountain where an elderly sage, pouring from a perpetual pot of tea, illustrated the advantages of cultivating a learner's mind. Had the young man heeded the sage and "emptied his cup," he might have found a remedy to the stresses of his long journey (and the burdens of his considerable ego) right in his own hands.

Thousands of years ago, in ancient China, Taoist sages noticed something that, today, Western medicine acknowledges: Stress can make us sick. Through study and experiment, these sages discovered that people under pressure develop energy blockages in their internal organs. In particular, when we internalize stress, the abdomen—the energetic center of the body and, as you'll recall, our primitive "gut brain"—becomes congested and cut off from other organs, such as the lungs and heart. Under stress, the nerves, blood vessels, and lymph nodes that cross paths in this region of the body become tangled and knotted, obstructing the flow of Qi and Blood and creating disharmonious weather that makes it difficult to attract the precious infant you so desire.

Thanks to our Taoist sages—and to modern-day teachers like Master Mantak Chia, founder of the *Universal Healing Tao,* who brought these ancient practices "down from the mountain"—you can do something about these knots, tangles, and blockages. Using a series of easy-to-master therapeutic techniques we refer to as internal organ acupressure, you can clear stormy abdominal weather in preparation for conception and pregnancy.

In the pages that follow, we'll explore three acupressure techniques that you and your partner can perform on yourselves or on each other to help restore your organs to harmony and health. You will learn to open your body's "wind gates," allowing healthful breezes to clear out congestion. You'll learn to restore the uterus to its natural place in the body in preparation for pregnancy. And women and men alike will learn to maintain the healthy flow of Blood and Qi to the organs that are vital to creating and carrying a baby.

GETTING TO KNOW YOU

If you've never performed acupressure on yourself before, you may feel a bit uncomfortable trying out these techniques.

Keep in mind that, in order to receive Quan Yin's gift of new life, you need to forge a very important new relationship in addition to the one you're working on with your partner. You need to love, respect, and *listen to* your body. It has much to tell you.

Before you try the acupressure techniques in this chapter, perform the following simple exercise. *Ladies, make sure you try this during the pre-ovulation stage of your cycle.*

Lie flat on a comfortable surface and close your eyes. Then, using your fingertips, slowly palpate the area around your navel. Be aware of every sensation you feel. Do some areas seem hard? Do others seem soft? Are certain places more sensitive than others?

Breathing comfortably and deeply, imagine that you are sending energy to your entire navel region, paying particular attention to sensitive spots. Imagine that your navel area is the perfect temperature—neither too warm nor too cool.

Congratulations—you've taken the first step toward getting to know the internal you. Now you're ready to build on that introduction!

COLD HANDS?

If you have a cooler constitution—including chilly extremities—you don't have to perform acupressure on your body with cold hands. To bring warmth to these important instruments of self-healing, try the technique we explored in "It's in Your Hands" on page 70. That way, when you touch your abdomen, you'll be contributing healing warmth, not taking it away.

OPENING YOUR WIND GATES

Remember the old saying "It's an ill wind that blows no good"? Traditional Chinese Medicine takes this idea to heart—or, I should say, to the belly.

In the Taoist view "winds" circulate inside your body, affecting your health and emotional life. These winds can enter from outside or emanate from inside. And if they become trapped in your body, these winds can become sick or stagnant—a definite sign of bad weather.

Think of your belly as the vortex where these many winds converge. Through that life portal in your middle—your navel—you can clear trapped winds and restore the healthy flow of Qi and Blood to all organs. You can breathe new life into your belly.

We call the acupressure technique you're about to learn Opening the Wind Gates. To perform it, you will press on points around the navel that correspond to specific internal organs. By pressing on these points, you can access and care for your organs without touching them directly.

Note that you may feel some discomfort while pressing certain points. Don't be concerned. That discomfort is simply alerting you to congestion in the corresponding organ, telling you to pay attention. When you feel tightness or discomfort, just press more gently, giving a little extra time to that point, breathing comfortably and deeply until the discomfort dissipates and you feel a change in the tissue under your fingers.

To understand the illustration above, think of the area around your navel as a clock, with 12 o'clock at the top of your navel. Starting at 3 o'clock, which

Opening the Wind Gates

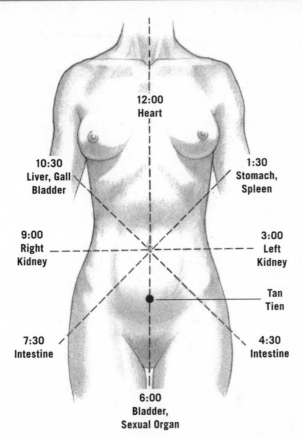

12:00
Heart

10:30
Liver, Gall
Bladder

1:30
Stomach,
Spleen

9:00
Right
Kidney

3:00
Left
Kidney

Tan
Tien

7:30
Intestine

4:30
Intestine

6:00
Bladder,
Sexual Organ

corresponds to your left kidney, you will press all the points counterclockwise around your navel, relieving congestion in the corresponding organs.

Ladies, take note: If you have not yet ovulated, perform the entire acupressure sequence that follows. If you are in the post-ovulation phase of your cycle (24 hours before ovulation until the first day of your next menstrual cycle, or through the first trimester if you become pregnant), I encourage you to perform this technique, but only above the abdomen. Do not open any of the wind gates below 3:00 and 9:00. This extra precaution will ensure the calmest internal weather possible, so that any fertilized eggs can implant in the uterus.

FEELING EMOTIONAL?

If you experience strong emotions while Opening the Wind Gates, don't be surprised. Your organs store memories of feelings you may have had many years ago. Opening the Wind Gates puts you in touch with these emotions, which helps you release old blockages that may have contributed to your infertility.

You can also manage powerful emotions by modifying the technique recommended to warm cold hands. (See "It's in Your Hands" on page 70.) After you have brought Qi to your hands, open your eyes and look around you. Then give yourself a task that takes you out of your emotions and into the material world: Look for objects of the same color or shape (for example, find all the red objects, or all the pointed objects). Concentrate on this task until you feel the wave of emotion subside.

Gentlemen: This practice, like others in this chapter, is a good remedy for Qi disharmonies that may be inhibiting your contribution to conception. It's also a good technique for maintaining total body health. I encourage you to make Opening the Wind Gates a regular part of your health care regimen.

1. Lie on your back, in bed or on the floor, with enough padding to be comfortable. Prop a pillow under your knees to support your lower back. Take a few breaths to relax before proceeding.

2. Awaken the energy in your abdomen by loosening the diaphragm, the large muscle that supports your lungs, just under your rib cage. Starting at the lower left corner of your rib cage (the side closest to your body's "exit," the rectum), gently press with the fingertips of both hands under your ribs toward your navel. Continue moving your fingers along, pressing toward your navel, until you reach the area just under your breastbone. Now move down the right of your rib cage, always pressing toward the navel, until you reach the lower right side of your rib cage. As you work on your diaphragm, inhale through your nose into your belly and exhale completely through your mouth.

3. Now move your attention to the "clock" around your navel. Starting at 3 o'clock, work just around the edge of your navel, along the slope where the skin rises from the navel to body level. Use your thumb or middle finger to apply pressure on each point until you feel a pulse.

4. Press the point in a tight spiral motion. If you notice any tightness or discomfort, change the direction of your spiral. As you press, breathe naturally, filling your belly with each inhalation through your nostrils, and exhaling through your mouth.

5. After three breaths (six breaths if you feel discomfort), stop pressing the point but continue to apply pressure. Use your mind to direct warmth and comfort to the corresponding organ.

6. Release and pause to let your energy settle before moving on to the next point.

7. Using the sequence shown in the illustration (1:30, stomach/spleen; 12:00, heart; and so on), travel counterclockwise around your navel, pressing and breathing at each point.

8. When you have completed the sequence, shake out your hands and feet gently to reinvigorate your extremities, stimulate your nerve endings, and activate your immune system.

 THE IMPORTANCE OF BELLY-BREATHING

Breathing from the belly—the body's center, the focal point for digestion and emotions, and the springboard for physical movement—is vital to Opening the Wind Gates. Belly-breathing slows you down, helps you stay connected with your body, and helps you relax fully. And by taking slow, deep and soft breaths, you fill your body with oxygen and clear it of stale air. So, as you Open the Wind Gates, be sure to inhale deeply and comfortably from your belly and exhale completely, tapping into the power of life-giving breath. Note that healthy belly-breathing is effortless; if you feel you're trying too hard, relax! Observe your belly as it rises and falls with each breath.

UTERUS LIFT

Ladies, you know where your uterus is. But do you know where it should be? Chances are, it resides a little lower in your body than it should.

Due to vertical, on-your-feet lifestyles; overheated constitutions; or diets that emphasize cold, raw foods and icy beverages, some 80 percent of women carry the uterus below its natural position in the body. Childbirth, which sometimes results in a prolapsed uterus; fibroids, which can weigh the uterus down; and other factors may also contribute to a low-placed uterus.

The acupressure technique you're about to learn—as old as Chinese medicine itself—can be used by any woman who's not pregnant, at any time in her life, to lift and strengthen her uterus. If you're preparing for pregnancy, consider it an important fertility enhancer and make it part of everyday life.

As you urinate—and I recommend you do this every time—clench your teeth to activate kidney energy* and press *out* with your bladder to force your urine stream. Then tighten the muscles in your pelvic floor (your PC muscle) to completely stop the flow of urine. (If you've ever done Kegel exercises to strengthen bladder control or enhance sexual response, you will be familiar with this technique.) Use your muscles to stop the flow of urine

The Uterus Lift Lying Down

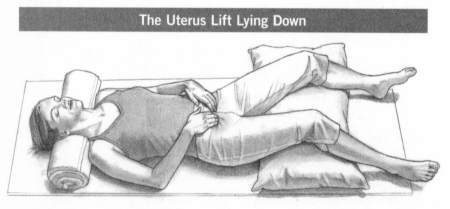

*In Traditional Chinese Medicine, the teeth are related to the kidneys and reproductive system, which are governed by the Water element. If we conjure kidney energy while urinating, we can strengthen both kidneys and teeth! Men, you can gain extra benefits by clenching your teeth and lifting your heels while urinating—strange, but true.

THE POWER OF NUMBERS

Numbers play an important role in Taoism and Traditional Chinese Medicine. Taoists believe the vibration of different numbers reflects the same energies that comprise the cosmos. For example, the number 36 is considered the perfect balance of Yang and Yin energies—3 representing Yang, 6 representing Yin. And the numbers 3, 6, and 9 represent the Three Treasures—Heaven, Human, and Earth—in congruency. So when the instructions in this book ask you to repeat an activity a certain number of times or hold a position for a certain number of seconds, know that you are not just fulfilling some whimsical requirement. You are synchronizing your body with the balanced, harmonious, congruent energies of the universe through the power of numbers.

three or more times until you have finished urinating. Now you're ready to lift your uterus:

1. Place the fingertips of both hands on the top of your pubic bone. (If you put your thumb on your navel and let your hand rest against your lower abdomen, your public bone should be near your little finger.)
2. Move your fingertips just above your pubic bone and press in toward your spine.
3. When you can't press any farther back toward your spine, your fingers will be under your uterus. Gently lift your uterus up toward your navel. Hold this position for 33 seconds, then release.

You can also perform the uterus lift at other times than when you are urinating—while standing, squatting, sitting, or lying down. If you are lying down, try this approach: Bend your knees and keep your feet flat. Put your fingers in position above your public bone. Inhale. Then, as you exhale, lower your knees by sticking out your heels as shown on opposite page; and lift your uterus, holding for 33 seconds before releasing.

GROIN PULSE ACUPRESSURE

Useful for both men and women, the groin pulse acupressure technique focuses on the reproductive system—clearing blockages in the femoral arteries and opening the vena cava, the large vein that allows Blood to flow from your legs to your reproductive organs and back again. In women, it's particularly helpful in bringing Blood and Qi to the uterus and ovaries, and in ensuring that both ovaries receive their fair share of vital essences. Gentlemen: You can think of the groin pulse acupressure technique as "nature's Viagra"—an easy way to improve bloodflow to the genitals. Men and women alike should perform this technique once or twice daily.

1. Lie on your back with your knees slightly bent and feet flat.
2. Place the fingertips of both hands on the top of your pubic bone. (If you put your thumb on your navel and let your hand rest against your lower abdomen, your pubic bone should be near your little finger.)
3. Slide your fingers out toward your legs until you reach the fold that separates your lower abdomen from your thighs as shown. Lightly palpate this area, feeling for a slight dip on each side. There you should feel a pulse.
4. Place a finger on each pulse. Notice how these pulses feel in relation to each other, paying attention to strength, intensity, speed, tension (hard or soft), and sensitivity (painful/achy or comfortable).
5. Using a rotating motion, apply pressure to the pulses with your fingers. Your goal is to use the pressure of your fingers to equalize strength, intensity, speed, tension, and sensitivity between the two pulses. If your rotations do not make a difference, apply more pressure to the weaker pulse, then hold the bloodflow for a count of 9 seconds.
6. When the pressures begin to equalize (meaning that strength, intensity, speed, tension, and sensitivity are balanced across both

Groin Pulse Acupressure

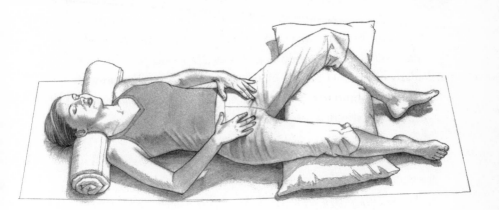

pulses), apply even pressure to both sides for 36 seconds. Imagine that you are closing the floodgates—building up pressure within both arteries.

7. Release the pressure by brushing your hands gently down the top of your inner thighs to allow the blood to flush down your legs. You may feel a warm or tingling sensation, which will happen more frequently with practice.

Michael and Melissa's Story
NOT TOO HIGH FOR HOPE

*L*ouise had her first hot flash at age 25 and was experiencing
night sweats so severe they soaked the sheets. Her periods started
coming further and further apart until they ceased altogether. At
first, Louise thought it was all in her head. Maybe it was stress?
After all, she had a busy career as an opera singer and traveled
frequently.

As her symptoms worsened, she sought a Western diagnosis. With
her FSH above 65—so high she was rejected from a National Institutes of Health study on infertility—specialists determined that she
was entering premature menopause, the result of an autoimmune
disorder in which antibodies attack the ovaries, causing premature
ovarian failure. When her doctor called to tell her the prognosis—
and that she might want to start shopping for an egg donor if she
wanted a child—she hung up the phone and sobbed.

A visit to an endocrinologist left Louise equally distressed. He
suggested she go on hormone replacement therapy, gave her the name
of an infertility support group, and wished her good luck. The entire
consultation lasted 15 minutes, she told me later.

Louise and I had once worked successfully together to address her
migraine headaches. So, when she received her tough infertility
diagnosis, she came back to our clinic. Following a program that
put tools for improving fertility in her hands—not just her doctor's—restored Louise's sense of control over her reproductive destiny. And, she said, she appreciated an approach that didn't simply
accept the finality of an FSH test.

We worked together to harmonize and balance Louise's body—
adding cooling foods to her diet, eliminating hot foods, and introducing the Six Healing Sounds (see page 123). Her hot flashes
became manageable, her period returned, and at age 30 she became

pregnant—delighted that the child she'd dreamed of had finally manifested.

Two years after the birth of her baby boy, Michael, Louise returned to our clinic. Her FSH had again risen, this time to 56. She began the Fertility Wisdom *program anew, sticking to its eating, drinking, and other guidelines. Within 2 months, she was pregnant again, with Melissa.*

Today, when Louise talks about her experiences, she has a seasoned perspective on Western fertility testing. FSH, she believes, can be a guide, but it's not an absolute measure of one's potential for conception. After all, in these many years, her FSH has never normalized; menstruating and ovulating have been rare occurrences. But, empowered by Traditional Chinese Medicine, Louise has two miracle babies to prove that what some deem impossible can be achieved when we choose to help ourselves.

CHAPTER 6

SMILE AND BREATHE: TAOIST MEDITATIONS

If you're feeling sad and wistful, what's a fast way to turn your attitude around? Smile at someone—even a stranger. And when you're overwhelmed and anxious, what's the best way to calm down quickly? I'll bet your answer is this: Sit quietly for a few minutes, breathing deeply and clearing your mind.

Ancient Taoist sages understood the power of these simple practices and used them as the foundation for the three meditations you'll find on the pages that follow. If you truly want to bring balance, harmony, and congruency to mind, body, and spirit—and improve your chances of conceiving—I invite you and your partner to make these meditations part of your life. Try them for just 1 month, and you'll be amazed at the improvements in your health and well-being.

INNER SMILE MEDITATION

In the 20th century, Western doctors began to acknowledge a correlation between health and happiness. Since that time, the annals of medical knowledge have come to include examples of people who cured life-threatening illnesses through laughter and a positive attitude. And a number of scientific studies have confirmed that smiling and positive emotions can heal both the spirit and the body. For example, a recent biofeedback study found that when you smile, your brain consumes only half the oxygen it usually requires, so the air you take in lasts twice as long. Another study has shown that achieving higher levels of consciousness such as joy, peace, and enlightenment leads to greater physical strength and healing. And yet another reveals that the electromagnetic field generated by your heart, the seat of smiling energy, can affect the energy of people around you—a good reason to smile to and appreciate your heart!

You can harness the healing power of happiness by mastering a special Taoist meditation we call the Inner Smile. It's simple: You smile to your organs and thank them for a lifetime of hard work in keeping your body operating. By tapping into the expansive energy of happiness, you will warm and heal your organs, relieve the effects of stress and tension, and create the inner openness and harmony necessary to attract new life.

You can do the Inner Smile in bed upon wakening or before going to sleep. (Many people find the Inner Smile especially helpful in the morning because it lifts energy.) If you've just eaten, wait at least 1 hour before you begin the Inner Smile.

Part 1 (see illustration on opposite page)

1. Sit at the edge of a chair with your back erect. Place your hands with the right palm on top of the left, in front of your navel. Close your eyes and breathe normally. Then proceed with the Inner Smile, parts 1 through 3.
2. Relax your forehead. Imagine meeting someone you love, or seeing a beautiful sight—perhaps the face of the baby you wish to welcome. Feel that smiling energy in your eyes.
3. Allow the smiling energy to flow to the midpoint between your eyebrows, then to your nose and cheeks. Feel it relaxing the skin on your face, then let it deeply warm your whole face. Let it flow into your mouth, and lift the corners of your mouth into a smile. Relax your jaw. Let your smile flow into your tongue. Then place the tip of your tongue on the roof of your mouth just behind your teeth and keep it there through the rest of the meditation.
4. Smile into your neck and throat, then into the front of your neck to your thyroid gland.

The Inner Smile

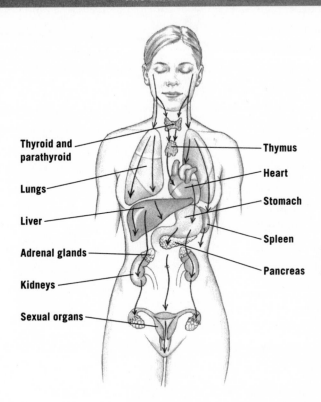

Thyroid and parathyroid

Lungs

Liver

Adrenal glands

Kidneys

Sexual organs

Thymus

Heart

Stomach

Spleen

Pancreas

5. Let the energy flow down to your thymus gland. Feel that gland grow bigger, like a bulb, and gradually blossom.

6. Let the energy from your thymus gland flow to your heart, and let it fill your heart with joy. Thank your heart for its hard work in circulating Blood throughout your body.

7. Continue by bringing the smile to your lungs, liver, kidneys, pancreas, and spleen, thanking each organ for its marvelous work.

8. Bring the smiling energy down to your genital area. Feel personal power and creativity. Let love, joy, kindness, and gentleness flow into your sexual organs.

The Inner Smile (cont.)

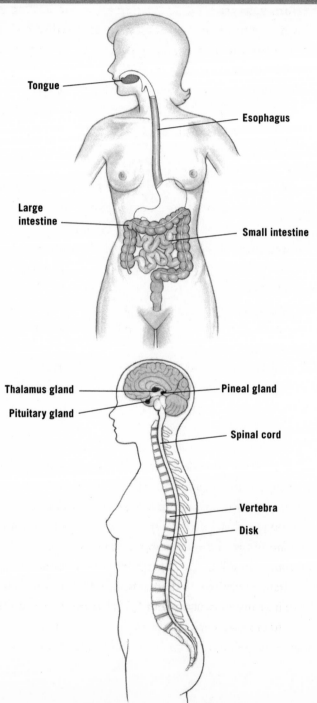

Part 2 (see illustration on opposite page)

9. Return your attention to your eyes. Let the smiling energy flow down to your mouth. Then build up some saliva by working your mouth around and swishing your tongue. Tuck your chin in. Swallow the saliva quickly, making a gulping sound.

10. Follow the saliva down through your digestive tract, smiling into your esophagus, small intestine, and large intestine, thanking each organ for its hard work in digesting your food and eliminating wastes.

Part 3 (see illustration on opposite page)

11. Bring the smiling energy back to your eyes. Smile inward, moving its power toward your third eye (middle eyebrow). Then direct the smile into your brain.

12. Smile into your pituitary, thalamus, and pineal glands, and thank them for their hard work. Move the smiling energy back and forth across your brain to balance the left and right sides and strengthen the nerves.

13. Move the smiling energy down through your brain and the back of your neck, then down to your spinal cord. Smile to each vertebra and disc.

14. Return the smiling energy to your eyes, and direct it quickly through your whole body in the same sequence as before. Feel the energy descend down your body like a shower or waterfall. Feel your whole body being loved and appreciated.

15. Concentrate the smiling energy in your navel area and mentally move it in an outward spiral around your navel 36 times, without going above the diaphragm or below the pubic bone. Women, start the spiral counterclockwise. Men, start it clockwise.

16. Reverse the direction of the spiral and circle it 24 times. Feel all your smiling energy stored below your navel like a round Qi ball. Think of your Qi ball as your energy savings account: Every time you meditate, image that you are refining that energy, then collect and store it below your navel. Your Qi ball is there for you whenever you need to tap your energy reserves.

17. Continue with the Microcosmic Orbit meditation, described next.

MICROCOSMIC ORBIT MEDITATION

As you learned in chapter 1, Qi flows through your body along invisible pathways called meridians. Two major energy channels connect these meridians to circulate Qi—the Functional Channel, which runs up the front of your body, and the Governor Channel, which runs down the back.

When you touch your tongue to the roof of your mouth just behind your front teeth, you connect these two channels to form a single circuit of energy, which Taoist sages called the Microcosmic Orbit. By using the Microcosmic Orbit meditation, you open up this vital energy channel to release blockages and revitalize and circulate Qi to all parts of your mind and body.

Each morning after you finish the Inner Smile meditation, sit quietly for a few moments. Connect with the Qi ball you stored below your navel at

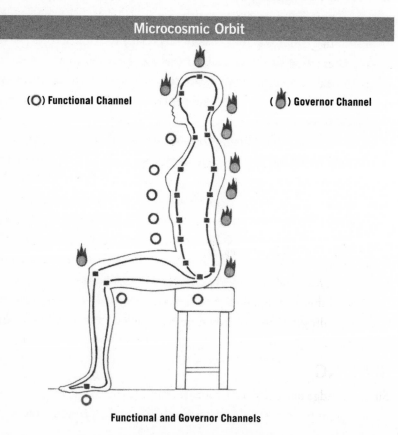

Microcosmic Orbit

(O) Functional Channel   ( ) Governor Channel

Functional and Governor Channels

the end of the Inner Smile. Then touch your tongue to the roof of your mouth and visualize a complete circle extending from the crown of your head down the front of your body to the tip of your toes, then up the back of your body and back to the crown of your head. This circle is the Microcosmic Orbit, try to experience the flow of Qi as a continuous current.

Now draw on the energy stored in your Qi ball and circulate it in the Microcosmic Orbit. Eventually the current should begin to feel warm in some places as it loops around. Continue to relax and let your mind flow with your Qi for a few minutes. Then gather the energy in your Qi ball for storage below your navel.

THE SIX HEALING SOUNDS

Traditional Chinese Medicine teaches that each organ is surrounded by a sac or membrane, called the fascia, which regulates that organ's temperature. Stress causes the membrane to stick to the organ, preventing the organ from releasing heat and exchanging it for cool energy. When this happens, the organ begins to overheat and the skin becomes clogged with toxins.

Credit Taoist sages for finding a way to release this trapped heat and toxicity. Centuries ago, during their meditations, they discovered that healthy organs vibrate at particular sound frequencies. They developed six sounds—we call them the Six Healing Sounds—that emulate those frequencies and combined them with postures that activate the acupuncture meridians of each organ. When the sounds and postures are performed in a particular sequence, heat given off by our organs is transferred out of the body through the esophagus. In the process, emotions such as anxiety, sadness, anger, fear, and worry—are cleared from our bodies.

Perform this technique at least once a day. As you'll see, you can practice the Six Healing Sounds while sitting, lying down, or even while walking. Here's how:

SITTING

Sit on the edge of a chair with your feet firmly planted on the ground, your back straight but comfortable, and your hands resting on your thighs, with palms up and fingers gently curved. As you assume the posture and make the sound for each organ—three, six, or nine times—keep your eyes open and your awareness centered on the part of your body you are healing. Do each movement slowly.

1. **Lungs:** Become aware of your lungs. Take a deep breath as you rotate your palms and bring them above your head elbows rounded. Look up, close your jaws, and part your lips slightly. Allow your breath to escape through the space between your teeth, making the sound *Sssss* (like a snake) subvocally, slowly and evenly, in one breath. Picture the color white, and see any excess heat and toxins in your lungs being released, as well as sadness and grief. When you have exhaled completely, bring your hands down and place them on your thighs, palms up. Then close your eyes, breathe normally, smile down to your lungs, and imagine the qualities of confidence and courage entering them.

2. **Kidneys:** Become aware of your kidneys. Take a deep breath as you bend forward and hook your hands around your knees. Pull on your arms from your lower back, being sure to round your back. Look straight ahead, round your lips, and subvocally make the sound *Whoooo,* as though you are blowing out a candle or imitating the wind. Picture the color blue, and see any excess heat and toxins in your kidneys being released, as well as fear and stress. When you have exhaled completely, release your hands and place them on your thighs, palms up. Sit up, close your eyes, breathe normally, smile down to your kidneys, and imagine the quality of gentleness and calmness entering them.

3. **Liver:** Become aware of your liver. Take a deep breath as you slowly swing your arms over your head and to the left. Interlace your fingers and, keeping your elbows straight, rotate your palms toward the ceiling and look at your hands. As you exhale, subvocally make the sound *Shhhh.* Picture the color green, and see any excess heat and toxins in your liver being released, as well as anger and frustration. When you have exhaled completely, release your hands and place them on your thighs, palms up. Sit up, close your eyes, breathe

normally, smile down to your liver, and imagine the qualities of tenderness and kindness entering it.

4. ***Heart:*** Become aware of your heart. Take a deep breath as you slowly swing your arms over your head and to the right, elbows straight. Interlace your fingers and rotate your palms toward the ceiling. As you exhale, open your mouth, round your lips, and subvocally make the sound *Haaaaw*. Picture the color red, and see any excess heat and toxins in your heart being released, along with any anxiety or impatience. When you have exhaled completely, release your hands and place them on your thighs, palms up. Sit up, close your eyes, breathe normally, smile down to your heart, and imagine the qualities of love and joy entering it.

5. ***Spleen:*** Become aware of your spleen. Take a deep breath as you place your index fingers at the bottom and slightly to the left of your sternum. Press in as you push your middle back outward. As you exhale, subvocally make the sound *Vvvvv* (making sure your upper teeth touch your lower lip). Picture the color yellow, and see any excess heat and toxins in your spleen being released, as well as worry and panic. When you have exhaled completely, release your hands and place them on your thighs, palms up. Sit up, close your eyes, breathe normally, smile down to your spleen, and imagine the qualities of fairness and openness entering it.

6. ***Triple Warmer**:** Lie on your back, close your eyes, and take a deep breath, inhaling into your chest, solar plexus, and lower abdomen. As you exhale, subvocally make the sound *Sheeee*. Imagine a large roller pressing out your breath along with

REMEMBER . . .
Sitting in traffic and stressed out? Do the Triple Warmer sound—*Sheeee*—subvocally and feel your tension dissipate.

---

*The triple warmer sound balances the temperature of the three energy centers of the body—the upper level, which includes the brain, heart, and lungs; the middle level, which includes the liver, kidneys, stomach, pancreas, and spleen; and the lower level, which includes the large and small intestines, bladder, and sexual organs. This sound is especially helpful at night in preparing for sleep.

any leftover toxins or excess heat as it moves from your head down to your feet. Now smile to all your organs. Imagine that your entire body is transparent—cleared of excess heat, toxins, and low-energy emotions.

LYING DOWN

After you've mastered the sounds, sitting postures, and visualizations of this practice, try it while lying down—it's a great way to spend a few moments in bed before you fall asleep. Follow the same basic instructions as for sitting, with these adjustments.

1. *Lungs:* Round your arms and raise them so that your elbows are at eye level above your head, with palms up and hands slightly apart. Now visualize the color white and exhale any trapped heat and toxins, grief, and sadness from your lungs: *Sssss.*

2. *Kidneys:* Just as you would while sitting, bring your knees toward your chest, stretching your lower back. Use your hands to hold your knees close to your chest. Now visualize the color blue and exhale any trapped heat and toxins and fear and stress from your kidneys: *Whoooo.*

3. *Liver:* Raise your arms above your head so that your right arm is extended and your left hand grasps your right elbow, creating a gentle stretch to the left. Now visualize the color green and exhale any heat, toxins, anger and frustration from your liver: *Shhhh.*

4. *Heart:* Raise your arms above your head so your hands meet in a point with your fingertips touching each other. Visualize the color red and exhale any trapped heat and impatience from your heart: *Haaaaw.*

5. *Spleen:* As in the sitting posture, place your index fingers at the bottom and slightly to the left of the sternum, pressing in as you push your middle back toward the floor or bed. Visualize the color yellow and exhale any heat and worry from your spleen: *Vvvvv* (with teeth touching lower lip).

6. *Triple Warmer:* Same as for sitting.

The Six Healing Sounds— Lying Down

Sssss

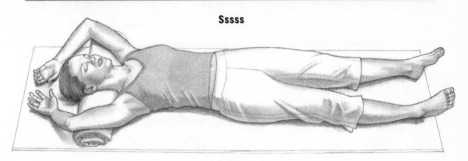

1. Lung Posture and Sound

Whooo

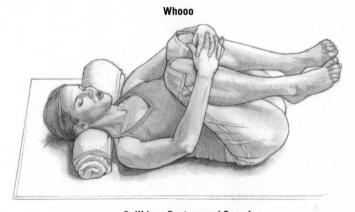

2. Kidney Posture and Sound

Shhhh

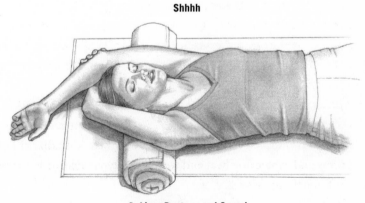

3. Liver Posture and Sound

(continued)

The Six Healing Sounds— Lying Down—cont.

Haaaaw

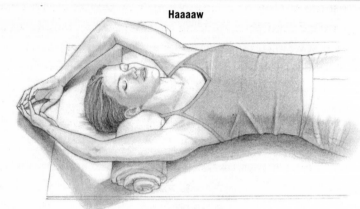

4. Heart Posture and Sound

Vvvvv

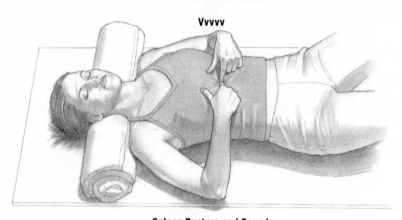

Spleen Posture and Sound

Sheeee

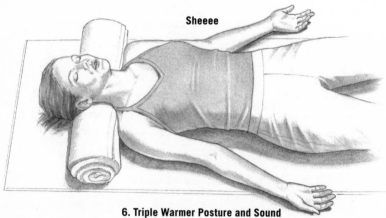

6. Triple Warmer Posture and Sound

WALKING

On my first trip to New York City, I was determined to see every famous sight, from the Empire State Building to Times Square. But, unfamiliar with East Coast weather, I had dressed for a typical San Francisco summer day (chilly fog rather than humid heat)—a choice I particularly regretted as my friends and I went below ground for the sweltering subway ride I insisted must be part of my New York experience. To keep cool, I did the Six Healing Sounds subvocally, on the subway and throughout the afternoon. At 2:00 a.m., when everyone else was limp and exhausted, I was cool, rested, and ready for more New York—and I thank the healing sounds.

You, too, can benefit from the healing sounds while you're on the go. Simply perform them subvocally, without the postures but in sequence, as you move. Do each sound three, six, or nine times, repeating the sequence until you feel rejuvenated. As you perform the sounds, be sure to smile to the organ you're cooling and healing.

CHAPTER 7

MOVE YOUR BODY: QI GONG EXERCISES

These days, it's hard to read a newspaper or magazine or visit any kind of health care provider without hearing about the benefits of exercise. Taoists have understood the connection between health and exercise for thousands of years. They believed that leading a sedentary life makes us forget how to live in our bodies, which eventually makes us forget who we really are. In fact, archaeologists have discovered ample evidence that calisthenics and breathing exercises were practiced in China as early as 1100 BC.

Over the centuries since that time, Taoists developed a meditative system of exercise called Qi Gong, which is now practiced around the world. Through prescribed movements, Qi Gong—which includes Tai Chi, a practice familiar to many—improves the circulation of Blood and Qi throughout the body, cultivating balanced, harmonious internal weather.

In the pages that follow, you will find a series of Qi Gong exercises for men and women that are especially beneficial to the reproductive system. These exercises can be practiced in a shorter period of time and a much smaller space than Tai Chi, yet they provide the same benefit of improved Qi flow.

Because healthy Qi is so important to male fertility—and so easily affected through activity—I recommend that men practice these exercises daily, women at least every other day. Ladies, please note any *Post-Ovulation Precautions* included with the exercises that follow; some of the exercises may be practiced throughout your menstrual cycle, others are best avoided after ovulation (in case you are pregnant) and during the first trimester of pregnancy because they engage the PC muscle. (As you'll recall, a tiny embryo needs calm and quiet to implant and thrive.) All of these exercises offer benefits when practiced during your period because they improve circulation.

Now it's time to get up and get active—and reap the rewards of Qi Gong!

FROM WARMUP THROUGH COOLDOWN

In chapter 4, I recommended that you start a meal with cooked, warming foods and end it with cooler foods so that your body is gently awakened to the process of digestion. Similarly, the Qi Gong exercises that follow start with warmups, then move to more intensive exercises once your body is awakened to movement, and conclude with a gentle and easy "cooldown."

Again, to realize the full benefits of these ancient and powerful techniques, I recommend that men make time to complete the entire sequence, from warmup through cooldown, every day—women at least every other day. (Although these exercises may seem like a lot at first, once you're familiar with them, it should take only about a half-hour to complete them all. And as you become more proficient, you'll notice more benefits!)

 A WORD OF CAUTION

Be sure to listen to your body as you practice these exercises. Your goal is to loosen your joints and relax your muscles so your Qi and Blood can flow freely. If you feel severe pain, back off until the exercise feels comfortable, or stop completely. Don't push yourself to your limits, especially at the beginning. And be sensitive to any injuries, chronic problems, or physical limitations you may have. If you're kind and gentle to your body, your body will start to trust you and relax. You'll find yourself gradually loosening up on a deeper level without having to force the issue. If you have injuries or any other health challenges, please consulta physician or other health specialist before undertaking these exercises.

To achieve the maximum benefits from your investment in Qi Gong, take the following steps after completing each individual exercise:

1. Remain still for a moment and bring your awareness to any sensations in your body.
2. Note any places where you feel discomfort or pain. Then bring "smiling energy"—starting with a smile on your face—to those places.
3. Observe how your breath fills your abdominal area.
4. To retain the benefit of the exercise you've just performed, imagine that you are gathering the healing energy in your navel. If you have a history of high blood pressure, visualize storing the energy lower— in your perineum, the area just in front of the anus (see the illustration on page 147). If you have a history of low blood pressure, store the energy higher—at your third eye, between your eyebrows.

WARMUP EXERCISES

The following 14 exercises are good for limbering and warming up your body before more intensive Qi Gong. They're best done in their entirety, in the sequence recommended, but if necessary, you can perform them separately or in groups according to any *Remember . . .* tip boxes included with the instructions.

~~~~ Energizer or Reverse Breathing ~~~~

Taoists call it Reverse Breathing because it's exactly the opposite of the way we usually breathe: Instead of expanding the trunk and abdomen to inhale and contracting to exhale, you contract to inhale and expand to exhale.

This is a good exercise for warming a cooler constitution. (Taoist sages would perform reverse breathing to stay warm in even the coldest outdoor weather, often wearing very little clothing!) If you have a warmer constitution, you can still do Energizer Breathing to warm up before Qi Gong

REMEMBER—BALANCE ACTIVITY WITH REST!

From a Taoist perspective, active exercise is just one ingredient in the formula for a healthy, harmonious, balanced, fertile body. For men and women alike, relaxation, meditation, and plenty of restful sleep are just as vital as exercise to preparing our bodies for conception and pregnancy—particularly if your internal weather is overheated. As you integrate these Qi Gong exercises into your life, consider the following:

- If your constitution is overheated (extreme morning thirst? red, cracked tongue? easily agitated?), take stock of your daily activities. Are you exercising too frequently or too vigorously? Are you balancing exercise with adequate rest? Are you drinking enough (room or body temperature) water and consuming enough healthy food to sustain your activity level? (People with warm constitutions should be eating more juicy foods to provide their bodies with enough fluid and using cooking methods that preserve the water content of food, such as steaming. People with cooler constitutions should choose denser foods, such as root vegetables, which generate more warmth as they are digested, and may use warmth-adding cooking methods.)

- Some people benefit most from Qi Gong in the morning because it energizes them for the day. Others prefer the evening, to relieve the stresses of the day. Experiment to determine which time of day works best for you.

- Intense exercise isn't the only activity that can tax our bodies and compromise our Qi. Many of us spend hours on our feet at work, hunched over the computer without taking a break, or on telephone conferences. Qi Gong exercises, balanced with Taoist meditations like the Inner Smile and Six Healing Sounds, plus good sleep, can help us put the stresses of these intensive activities behind us.

- I cannot emphasize it enough: *If you are a woman in the second phase of your cycle—post-ovulation, when pregnancy is possible—or if you are in the first trimester of your pregnancy, curtail all rigorous physical activity for the time being.* A gentle walk on a flat surface can be good for your body and the baby you are or might be carrying. Gentle stretching is also beneficial. Biking, hiking, intensive swimming and yoga, even walking up flight after flight of stairs—or any other activity that engages your PC muscle—aren't appropriate now.

exercises; just be sure your daily regimen also includes plenty of Healing Sounds to release excess heat and toxicity from your body.

Here's how it's done.

1. Stand or sit comfortably.

2. Breathe rhythmically and fairly quickly, but not so fast that you become dizzy! Flatten your abdomen and contract your trunk cavity as you inhale and expand it as you exhale. To start, breathe both in and out only through your nostrils.

> **REMEMBER . . .**
> You can perform Energizer Breathing by itself, perhaps in the morning, and particularly in winter, or whenever you need to warm up and energize your body quickly.

3. Repeat 9, 18, or 27 times. After completing the exercise, take a moment to "gather" the energy you've created by imagining it spiraling nine times clockwise, then nine times counterclockwise around your navel.

4. When you've mastered the technique, you can inhale through your nose and exhale through your mouth.

~~~~~ Laughing Qi Gong ~~~~~

This exercise may be performed while standing, lying down, or sitting. To start, take a few deep breaths and relax your body.

1. Bring your attention to your thoracic cavity (your chest area), particularly to your heart and lungs. (If you like, you may place your hands on your sternum, or breastbone.) Now, take a deep breath, and as you exhale, laugh loudly, *with your mouth open,* as though you've just heard the funniest joke in the world. Let your chest shake vigorously as you laugh. Repeat for three inhalation/exhalation cycles.

2. Bring your attention to your abdominal cavity, or solar plexus, midway between your sternum and navel. (You may place your

hands on either side of your rib cage if you like.) Now, take a deep breath and expand your rib cage; then, as you exhale, laugh—a hearty chuckle—*with your mouth closed*. Let your abdominal cavity shake as you laugh. Repeat for three inhalation/exhalation cycles.

> **REMEMBER . . .**
> Laughing Qi Gong is one of the warmup exercises that engage your whole body. It can be performed alone, in conjunction with Loosening the Waist and Opening the Door of Life, or as part of the entire Qi Gong sequence.

3. Bring your attention to your lower abdomen, just above your pubic bone. Taoists call this area the Ovarian Palace in women and the Sperm Palace in men. (Place your hands there if you like.) Now, take a deep breath and, as you exhale, squeeze your PC muscle and laugh *subvocally* as though you've just heard something amusing. Let your lower abdomen shake gently as you laugh. Repeat for three inhalation/exhalation cycles.

4. Now bring the laughing energy from your chest, solar plexus, and Ovarian or Sperm Palace into your navel. (Visualize a spot right in the center of your body, midway between your navel and spine.) Now, visualizing a circle about 3 inches in diameter, with your navel at the center, spiral the laughing energy clockwise nine times, then counterclockwise nine times, retaining the laughing energy there.

~~~~~Loosening the Waist~~~~~

1. Stand with your feet parallel to each other, slightly wider than shoulder-width apart. Allow your arms to dangle loosely at your sides. Begin to turn your hips from side to side. Let your arms swing naturally and easily with the momentum of your turning hips. Explore your natural and comfortable range of hip motion in this way. Don't go to extremes; just stay within your free and easy comfort zone.

2. After turning just your hips 10 or 12 times, allow your lumbar vertebrae to relax and loosen and gently twist with the motion.

You should still begin the movement from your hips, but allow
the lumbar vertebrae to respond.

3. Next allow your middle spine,
    upper back, and neck to twist
    gently with the movement. Keep
    your shoulders loose and let your
    arms swing as you move. Don't
    use effort to move your arms; let
    them be totally limp and just let
    your body swing them. At the same time, be aware of the gentle
    twisting of your knee and ankle joints as you twist your whole
    body.

4. Do this at least 36 times to each side.

> **REMEMBER . . .**
>
> Loosening the Waist may be
> performed alone, in
> conjunction with Laughing Qi
> Gong and Opening the Door
> of Life, or as part of the
> entire Qi Gong sequence.

～～～Opening the Door of Life ～～～

1. Begin in the same stance as for
    Loosening the Waist. Twist to the
    left as in the previous exercise,
    initiating the movement from your
    hips. Let your right arm swing
    across the front of your torso,
    raising it up to head height with
    your palm facing away from you.
    At the same time, let your left arm
    swing around to the back and place the back of your left hand over
    the Door of Life—the point on the spine opposite the navel.

> **REMEMBER . . .**
>
> Opening the Door of Life may
> be performed alone, in
> conjunction with Laughing Qi
> Gong and Loosening the
> Waist, or as part of the entire
> Qi Gong sequence.

2. When you reach your full extension, relax, and then extend again by
    loosening your lower back. Feel the gentle stretch and increased
    extension all the way from the Door of Life, not from the shoulders.
    Extend in this way two or three times.

3. Twist to the right and repeat the previous two steps on the right side.
    Repeat nine times on each side.

～Windmill: Opening the Spinal Joints ～

The Windmill exercise, designed to open all your spinal joints, has five phases. Do each phase very slowly and with awareness.

PHASE I: STRETCHING THE OUTER FRONT

REMEMBER . . .

The following four exercises (Windmill, Hip Rotations, Knee Rotations, and Ankle/Knee/Hip Rotations and Joint Opening) require greater concentration and should be done together or as part of the entire Qi Gong sequence.

1. Begin in the same stance as for Loosening the Waist. Bring your hands together and hook your thumbs together. Keeping your hands close to your torso, inhale and raise your arms until they are extended straight up over your head, with fingers pointing upward. Gently stretch up in this position, extending your spine slightly backwards. You can even say *Ahhhhh* as you would when you stretch first thing in the morning.

2. Begin to exhale slowly and bend forward, reaching as far out in front as you can, keeping your head between your arms. Try to feel each joint of your spine releasing one by one in a wavelike motion. Bend first from the lumbar vertebrae (lower/mid back), then from the thoracic vertebrae (upper back/chest), and finally from the cervical vertebrae (neck). At this point, you are bent all the way over.

3. Slowly straighten back up, again feeling each joint of your spine opening, all the way from your sacrum (the large bone at the base of your spinal column, located above your tailbone) up to the base of your neck. Let your arms and head hang heavily until you are back in the starting position. Repeat three to five times. Finish with your arms over your head as at the end of step 1.

PHASE II: STRETCHING THE INNER FRONT

1. Now do the same movements, but in reverse. Point your fingertips downward and slowly lower your arms, keeping your hands close to

your torso. When your arms are completely lowered, begin to bend forward; release your head, cervical vertebrae (neck), thoracic vertebrae (chest), and lumbar vertebrae (lower back), until you are bent all the way forward as at the end of step 2 of Phase I. Feel each joint opening.

2. Keeping your head between your arms, start to straighten up. Your arms will extend out in front as you slowly stand erect. When you finish straightening up, your arms will be straight up above your head. Repeat three to five times.

PHASE III: BENDING THE LEFT SIDE

1. Keeping your head between your arms in the overhead position, lean to the left. You should feel a gentle stretch on the left side of your waist. Continue stretching down and to the side until you are all the way down.

2. Circle back up on your right side until you are again standing straight with your arms overhead. Repeat three to five times.

PHASE IV: BENDING THE RIGHT SIDE

Repeat the same side-bending movements as in Phase III, but to the right. Do three to five times.

PHASE V: CONCLUSION

To finish, unhook your thumbs and let your arms slowly float back down to your sides.

Hip Rotations

1. Stand with your feet parallel and slightly wider than your shoulders. Place your hands on the sides of your waist. As you rotate your hips, keep your head above your feet. Move slowly and easily, breathing deeply and continuously.

2. Bring your hips forward.
3. Move your hips in a big circle to the right.
4. Now move your hips in a circle to the back.
5. Move your hips to the left.
6. Repeat steps 2 through 5 eight more times.
7. Reverse direction and repeat a total of nine times.

REMEMBER . . .
Perform Hip Rotations in conjunction with the Windmill, Knee Rotations, and Ankle/Knee/Hip Rotations and Joint Opening, or as part of the entire Qi Gong sequence.

Knee Rotations

1. Place your feet together. Bend your knees and place your palms lightly on your kneecaps.
2. Slowly and gently rotate your knees to the left.
3. Rotate your knees to the back.
4. Rotate your knees to the right.
5. Repeat steps 1 through 4 eight more times.
6. Now reverse direction and repeat nine times.

REMEMBER . . .
Perform Knee Rotations in conjunction with the Windmill, Hip Rotations, and Ankle/Knee/Hip Rotations and Joint Opening, or as part of the entire Qi Gong sequence.

Ankle/Knee/Hip Rotations and Joint Opening

1. Raise your right leg. With your hands on your hips, begin to rotate your right ankle 9 to 36 times clockwise, and then the same number of times counterclockwise.
2. Next, keeping the same leg raised, rotate your foreleg from the knee in

REMEMBER . . .
Perform Ankle/Knee/Hip Rotations and Joint Opening in conjunction with the Windmill, Hip Rotations, and Knee Rotations, or as part of the entire Qi Gong sequence.

a circular motion 9 to 36 times clockwise and then the same number of times counterclockwise.

3. Now, keeping the same leg raised, rotate the entire leg from the hip joint in a circular motion 9 to 36 times clockwise and then the same number of times counterclockwise.

4. Repeat steps 1 through 3 using your left leg.

~~~~Hitting the Tan Tien ~~~~

Post-Ovulation Precaution: This exercise is vigorous and/or engages the PC muscle. Ladies: Do not perform it during the second half of your cycle (post-ovulation) or during the first trimester of pregnancy.

REMEMBER . . .

May be performed alone, in conjunction with Bouncing and Shaking the Joints, or as part of the entire Qi Gong sequence.

1. Relax your arms completely, and gracefully swing them in free fall from left to right. As you swing to the left, your right hand should come in front of your body, with your palm hitting your navel area at the exact same time that the back of your left hand hits the Door of Life (on the back opposite the navel).

2. Then, as you swing to the right, your left hand comes in front of your body, with your palm hitting your navel area at the exact same time as the back of your right hand hits the Door of Life.

3. Repeat 36 times to each side.

~~~~Bouncing and Shaking the Joints ~~~~

Post-Ovulation Precaution: This exercise is vigorous and/or engages the PC muscle. Ladies: Do not perform it during the second half of your cycle (post-ovulation) or during the first trimester of pregnancy.

REMEMBER . . .

May be performed alone, in conjunction with Hitting the Tan Tien, or as part of the entire Qi Gong sequence.

1. Relax your body while concentrating on opening your joints, and bounce on the floor without any tension.

2. Let the vibration in your heels work its way up through your entire skeletal system, from legs to spine to neck to skull. Your shoulders and arms should vibrate as they hang loosely at the sides of your body. To enhance this, you can hum a vowel to hear the vibration make your voice tremble as well.

3. Rest and feel the Qi entering your joints.

~~~Dog Holding Leg: Opening the ~~~ Spinal Joints

1. Crouch with your knees bent and back curved. Your chest should not be touching your thighs. Now wrap your right arm around your right leg, with your left arm between your legs and clasping your right forearm near the elbow.

2. Now, while slowly pulling up, arch your back and feel the energy flowing through your spine and legs into the earth.

3. Repeat on the opposite side.

4. Now, bend your knees a little more and wrap both arms around both legs, clasping your right arm at the forearm with your left hand. Again, pull up as if you are lifting yourself, arching your back to facilitate the flow of energy throughout your skeletal system.

REMEMBER . . .
May be performed alone, in conjunction with the Spinal Alignment exercises, or as part of the entire Qi Gong sequence.

~~~Standing Spinal Alignment ~~~

1. Stand against a wall with your feet parallel and shoulder-width apart. Your spine should touch the wall. Relax your lower back or sacrum—the large bone at the base of your spinal column, located

Dog Holding Leg Posture

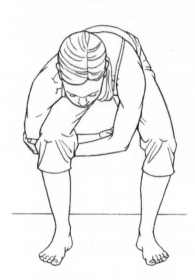

1.

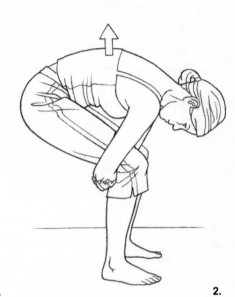

2.

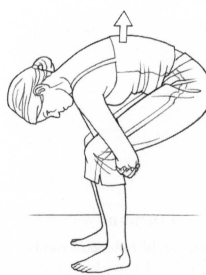

3.

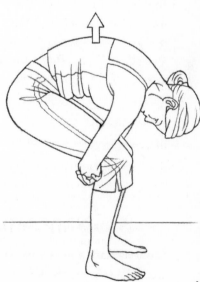

4.

above your tailbone.

2. Press your feet into the ground. Bend you knees slightly so that your knees are over your toes. Now, square your hips, and press your sacrum to the wall. Hold for a while, then relax. Feel the Qi flow up to your sacrum.

> **REMEMBER . . .**
>
> May be performed alone; with Dog Holding Leg and Aligning Your Spine with the Floor, in the order shown; or as part of the entire Qi Gong sequence.

3. Press your T-11 vertebra* against the wall. Hold for a while and relax. Feel the Qi flow up to your sacrum and T-11.

4. Now, sink your breastbone (sternum), pull in your chin and shoulder blades (scapulae), and bring your C-7 vertebra** close to the wall. Hold for a while and relax. Feel the Qi flow up through your sacrum, T-11, and C-7.

～Aligning Your Spine with the Floor ～

1. Lie on the floor. Feel your spine touching the ground. Draw both knees up and place feet flat on the ground, in parallel position.

> **REMEMBER . . .**
>
> May be performed alone; with Dog Holding Leg and Standing Spinal Alignment, in the order shown; or as part of the entire Qi Gong sequence.

2. Press your feet to the ground and feel your sacrum, spine, and head moved by your feet. Repeat a few times, and observe how your feet can move your whole body. Relax and feel the Qi flow.

---

*The 11th thoracic vertebra (T-11) is also called the adrenal center due to its close proximity to the adrenal glands. A good way to find T-11 is to find the point midway between the bottom of the sternum and the navel in front; we call this the solar plexus point. Draw your finger around to the point on the spine opposite the solar plexus; this is T-11. If you put your hand on this point and lean forward, you'll notice that it protrudes more than any other surrounding vertebrae.

**C-7 is the seventh and lowest cervical vertebra. The Chinese name for C-7, Ta Chui, means "big vertebra." It is the big bone at the base of the neck.

3. Now, press your feet to the ground. Press your sacrum and T-11 vertebra to the ground. Feel the sacrum and T-11 touching the ground and feel the alignment. Extend both arms, sink your chest, pull in your chin, and feel the C-7 point touch the ground. Relax and feel the Qi flow.

～～～～Bone Marrow Inner Smile～～～～

After completing the other exercises, stand for a while and smile to your entire skeletal structure. Take time to smile to each bone one by one.

1. Smile to your skull.
2. Smile to each cervical vertebra. Feel the Qi penetrate into each cervical vertebra, filling and expanding the space between vertebrae.
3. Smile to your collarbone all the way down to the bones of your wrists and hands—past your scapulae (shoulder blades), humerus (the bone that runs from shoulder to elbow), radius (from inside elbow to thumb), and ulna (from outside elbow to little finger). Smile especially to the joints between the bones; feel the Qi filling the joint space.
4. Smile down to your thoracic vertebrae, lumbar vertebrae, and pelvis. Feel the Qi filling and expanding the joint space.
5. Smile down to your groin and feel the Qi fill up the hip joint. Smile to your femur (thigh bone)—one of the major bones responsible for producing red blood cells.
6. Continue smiling down to your knee joint, and feel the joint fill with Qi; smile to the bones in your lower leg—the tibia and fibula—and the bones and joints of your ankles and feet.
7. Rest a moment and feel Qi flow through your entire skeletal structure. Then collect the energy in your Qi ball for storage below your navel.

Anna's Story
THE HEALING POWER OF MOVEMENT

*T*ory was a massage therapist when she began an internship at our clinic to learn more about the role of bodywork in Traditional Chinese Medicine. As we worked together at the clinic, Tory's personal story unfolded: Diagnosed with blocked Fallopian tubes, she had already undergone two in vitro fertilization cycles in an effort to conceive, and the failed procedures had left her discouraged, even bitter. Was there any hope for her through Traditional Chinese Medicine?

A thorough investigation of Tory's history and health revealed an extremely challenged constitution. Her tongue was very greasy-looking—an indicator of severe internal heat and dampness. And as I listened to Tory's tale, I noticed something else: Although Tory was sensitive when it came to helping others, when she talked about herself, her language was negative and critical.

I knew from experience that Tory could not truly heal others or welcome the baby she desired until she had healed herself. As she worked to make our Fertility Wisdom part of her life, Tory paid special attention to the Taoist meditations and Qi Gong exercises that could help her transform negative emotions into healing energy. As she learned to move her body in ways that cooled her warm constitution and facilitated the flow of Qi and Blood, Tory's attitude began to change.

Good health brought new hope. And after several months of preparation, Tory scheduled another IVF cycle for May, with a trip to Hawaii in April to ensure that she was fully relaxed and rested before the procedure. But when Tory and her husband returned from Hawaii, they brought more than souvenirs and new hope for their next IVF cycle. They also brought Anna—conceived in the islands but welcomed long before, when her mother discovered the healing power of movement.

The Perineum: The Qi Muscle

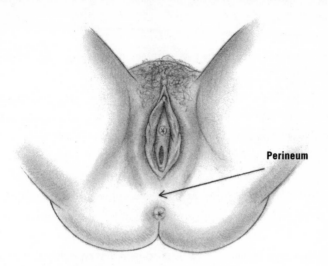

Perineum

INTENSIVE QI GONG

TAPPING PERINEUM POWER

One of the main objectives of Taoist Qi Gong is to boost the flow of Qi in the body. You will find one of your most important tools for achieving this goal right where you are sitting—in your perineum (see the illustration), which Taoists call the Qi muscle.

We call the perineum region, which includes the anus and sexual organs, the seat of Yin—the lowest point on the trunk where Yin energy collects, closely connected to all your organs and glands. Located between your body's two main gates—the front gate, through your sexual organs; and the back gate, through your rectum—the perineum is also known as the Gate of Death and Life.

A strong perineum is critical to keeping life force energy from leaking out the front gate and depleting the function of your sexual organs—including the ability to conceive and carry a baby.

In Taoist theory, the perineum or Qi muscle functions something like a pump. It is controlled through the PC muscle of the pelvic and urogenital floor, the sphincter muscle of the anus, and the many involuntary muscles located in the perineum region. By flooding this area with energy—which we can do through the breathing exercises that follow—we strengthen the perineum's ability to pump Qi up toward our internal organs and prevent it from leaking out. In short, we can train the perineum to tighten, close, and draw Qi back up your spine.

To understand how the perineum works, note that the anus region is divided into five sections—middle, front, back, left, and right. Each section is connected with different organs and glands. (See "How the Gate of Death and Life Is Connected to the Organs" on page 145.)

You can strengthen your Qi muscle and tap its power to preserve fertility as it preserves Qi by becoming aware of and appreciating its unique function and by doing what you'd do to strengthen any muscle: exercise it. (As with any exercise, the more you practice, the better you'll become at isolating and exercising your Qi muscle—and the stronger that muscle will become.)

1. Sit or stand comfortably. Inhale and exhale three deep breaths in preparation.
2. Now exhale quickly three times, expelling the air until your abdomen is flat. Keep your abdomen flat through the next four steps of this exercise.
3. Press your left foot into the floor. Inhale quickly three times, sniffing through your nose, while contracting the *left* side of your perineum/anus.
4. Press your right foot into the floor. Now, inhale quickly three times, sniffing through your nose, while contracting the *right* side of your perineum/anus.
5. Press your toes into the floor. Now, inhale quickly three times, sniffing through your nose, while contracting the *front* of your perineum/anus.
6. Press your heels into the floor. Now, inhale quickly three times, sniffing through your nose, while contracting the *back* of your perineum/anus.
7. Maintain this posture and hold your breath for as long as you are comfortable. Then exhale through your mouth.

HOW THE GATE OF DEATH AND LIFE IS CONNECTED TO THE ORGANS

Taoists call the perineum the Gate of Death and Life. To understand the perineum's relationship with other parts of the body, think of the anus region as divided into five sections—middle, front, back, left, and right. As this chart shows, by activating different sections of the anus, we can send healing energy to different organs.

ACTIVATE THIS SECTION OF THE ANUS	SEND HEALING ENERGY TO THESE ORGANS
Middle	Vagina and uterus; aorta and vena cava; stomach; heart; thyroid, parathyroid, pituitary, and pineal glands; top of the head
Front	Bladder; cervix; small intestine; stomach; thymus; thyroid; front part of brain
Back	Sacrum; lower lumbars; 12 thoracic vertebrae; 7 cervical vertebrae; small brain (cerebellum)
Left	Left ovary; large intestine; left kidney; left adrenal gland; spleen; left lung; left hemisphere of the brain
Right	Right ovary; large intestine; right kidney; right adrenal gland; liver; gall bladder; right lung; right hemisphere of the brain

8. Take three deep breaths through your nose, then shake out your hands and feet.

OVARIAN BREATHING—FOR WOMEN

Post-Ovulation Precaution: *This exercise is vigorous and/or engages the PC muscle. Ladies: Do not perform it during the second half of your cycle (post-ovulation) or during the first trimester of pregnancy.*

If you are a woman trying to get pregnant, you've probably already done some thinking about your ovaries. Are they healthy and functioning properly? Are they capable of producing viable eggs? It's time now to release any worries or fears you might have about the condition of your ovaries and do something to appreciate and help them, guided by the healing wisdom of Taoism.

Taoists observed that the ovaries play a very important role in the health of the human female. They not only produce the hormones and eggs required for reproduction, they also require the contributions of every other organ in the body to perform their functions. In short, the greater the energy reserves of the body's other organs, the healthier the ovaries; taxed or depleted organs have less Qi to share with the ovaries. (That's why it's so important to improve whole-body balance and harmony in order to boost a woman's fertility.)

Because ovaries store a woman's Yang energy—the energy of creation—they are great repositories of warmth. What's more, Taoists noted that ovaries have a special kind of Qi, denser than the Qi of other organs. Because ovarian energy moves more slowly than other body energy, we can improve fertility by ensuring that ovarian energy circulates effectively.

You can awaken and circulate ovarian energy by mastering an ancient technique called Ovarian Breathing. In this exercise you will draw the warm, dense, Yang energy of the ovaries into your perineum (your body's Qi pump), up your spine, and into your abdomen for storage. As with all Taoist practices, the more frequent your practice, the easier and more beneficial your practice will be!

You may perform Ovarian Breathing while sitting, standing, or lying down.

IF YOU SIT . . .

- Sit on the edge of a chair, feet shoulder's-width apart, using both your legs and your buttocks to stabilize and support your body. (Sit forward in order to avoid putting pressure on your sciatic nerve.) As you sit on the edge of the chair, your vagina and perineum should be unobstructed but covered with comfortable underwear or loose clothing to protect them from drafts. (To enhance the effect as ancient Taoist women did, you may wish to place a hard, round object, such as a ball, in such a way that it presses directly on the vagina and clitoris during practice, or you can sit on the heel of one foot, tightly

pressing the heel against the clitoris to help activate the Qi.)
- Unless you are sitting on one foot, plant both feet firmly on the ground. Keep your back straight at the waist but slightly round at the shoulders and neck. Your hands may be clasped gently in front of you or resting palms-up on your knees.

IF YOU STAND . . .

- Stand straight and relaxed, feet shoulder's-width apart, with your knees bent and your hands at your sides. (Be sure you are relaxed or Qi may become trapped in your heart area and cause irritability.)

IF YOU LIE DOWN . . .

- Lie on your right side with a pillow raising your head about 3 or 4 inches so that it sits squarely on your shoulders. Place the four fingers of your right hand immediately in front of your right ear, with the thumb behind the ear and folded slightly forward to keep your ear open. (It's important not to close your ear's Eustachian tube so that pressure may be balanced between both ears during Ovarian Breathing.)
- Rest your left hand on your outer left thigh.
- Keep your right leg straight; your left leg, which rests on the right, is slightly bent. (Ancient Taoists noted that this is the position in which animals often sleep. With their wise instincts, perhaps animals realize that this position relieves their spines from stress?)

Now, Ovarian Breathing, step by step:

1. Whichever posture you choose, raise your tongue to the roof of your mouth to open the Microcosmic Orbit, as you did in chapter 6.
   If you feel tense, do some gentle stretches or practice the Inner Smile meditation on page 117 to help yourself relax.
2. Find your Ovarian Palace by placing both thumbs at your navel and forming a triangle with your index fingers. Spread your little fingers so that they rest on your abdomen where your ovaries would be. Rub the ovaries to warm and awaken them.

3. Using very little pressure on your PC muscle, close and open your vagina to generate energy. Exhale quickly three times through your mouth. Inhale a short sip of air through your nose to bring more energy to the Ovarian Palace.

4. Take another sip of air and contract the outer and inner lips of the vagina to bring the ovarian energy down toward the perineum. Then bring the energy to the front of your perineum by contracting it.

5. Exhale and breathe normally. Then guide the warm energy from your ovaries back down toward your perineum, through the uterus, the cervical wall, and the back wall of the vagina.

6. Keeping your attention on your perineum, inhale and exhale nine times to build up more energy. Exhale completely to flatten your abdominal area. Then, keeping your tummy flat, inhale in short sniffs to draw the warm ovarian energy to your perineum again. By pulling up the middle and back of the perineum, draw the energy up to your coccyx, at the bottom of your spine. Tilt your sacrum by tipping your lower back slightly as if you were flattening it against a wall. Then tilt the sacrum downward and hold it in this position, maintaining the energy in the sacrum for a while. Imagine a miniature Sun flooding your entire abdominal area with pleasing warmth. Store this warm energy in your abdomen as you complete the Ovarian Breathing exercise.

7. Exhale through your mouth and relax. Then breathe normally, mindful of the warm, creative energy you have just generated.

COOL DOWN

~~~~~~~~~~~~~Monkey Dancing~~~~~~~~~~~~~

1. After completing your Qi Gong exercises, lie on your back on the floor. Relax and breathe for a moment.

2. Raise your arms and legs in the air.

REMEMBER . . .
Besides providing a cooldown after Qi Gong, this is a good exercise to perform after Opening the Wind Gates (see page 106), while you are still lying down.

TAPPING THE SUN'S HEALING WARMTH—FOR WOMEN WITH COOLER CONSTITUTIONS

If you have a warmer constitution, you will want to avoid spending time in the sun in order to cool your body. But if you are a woman whose constitution is cooler, let me share a Taoist secret that can bring healing warmth to your body. We call it *sunbathing,* but—unlike in Western culture—it has nothing to do with getting a tan. It's about bringing the creative, Yang energy of the sun to a part of your body that needs it when you're trying to conceive: your reproductive organs.

To sunbathe Taoist-style, find a comfortable place to lie down in the sun. Be sure you are wearing enough clothing to avoid drafts and to protect your skin from sunburn. For the greatest benefits from a Taoist perspective (and to avoid the sun's harshest rays), do this prior to 11:00 a.m., and for no more than 15 minutes. And *practice it only in the pre-ovulation phase of your cycle. As you perform this exercise, imagine that wour body is a miniature sun.*

1. First you will warm your Yang side, your back: Lie down on your belly with your buttocks directly facing the sun so that the lower portion of your body feels the sun's rays. (For comfort, you may put a pillow or blanket under your belly.) Place your arms above your head with your thumbs touching each other, keep your legs straight, and arch your feet so that your toes are touching the ground. (Your entire body, viewed from above, should look like a straight line—a Yang symbol.) Remain in this position, enjoying the warmth of the sun, for 9 minutes. Then turn over.

2. Now you will warm your Yin side, your belly: Lying on your back, bend your knees and let them fall to the sides, bringing the bottoms of your feet together (be sure your feet are touching). Lie so that you can feel the sun's warmth on your lower tummy and genital area. Place your hands under your lower back, with your thumbs touching each other. (Your body, viewed from above, should look like a circle—a Yin symbol.) Enjoy the warmth of the sun in this position for 6 minutes.

3. After sunbathing, drink a little water that is room temperature or warm-

3. Now shake out your hands and feet to stimulate the nerve endings in your extremities and activate your immune system.

4. You can also shake out your hands and feet while standing or sitting.

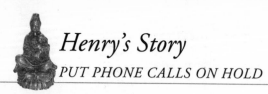

Henry's Story
PUT PHONE CALLS ON HOLD

*S*mart *and hardworking, Judith asked a lot of questions when she first came to our clinic. After one attempt at intrauterine insemination and a miscarriage, she was determined to do everything right for her future baby—and she wasn't taking any chances.*

Judith committed herself fully to Traditional Chinese Medicine and to bringing her body, with its cooler constitution, into harmony. She followed my advice to conserve precious vital energy by cutting back on her nonstop schedule and stressful work, including hours and hours of phone calls each day.

When she found out she was pregnant, Judith was ecstatic. But the memory of her miscarriage cautioned her to hold back. She decided not to tell anyone about the baby until a sonogram showed a healthy pregnancy. Then she could celebrate.

Although her sonogram revealed no complications, I began to notice the subtle erosion of Judith's vitality as her pregnancy progressed. She seemed to be leaking energy. After some prompting, she confessed that she was exhausted, and spotting. Despite my cautions, she had reverted to her pre-pregnancy lifestyle, including marathon phone calls—an activity that, because it involves sitting, gives the false appearance of being "relaxing." (From an Eastern perspective, every time you open your mouth to speak, you're using precious Qi that could be sustaining your pregnancy.)

After some strict coaching, I persuaded Judith to put the phone on hold while the seed inside her grew. Her spotting diminished. Her vitality returned. And her perseverance paid off when, after three short pushes, she delivered Henry, healthy as could be. Six months later, Judith was back in our clinic, preparing her body for the one ambition she is not ready to put on hold: her second child (which turned out to be a girl).

CHAPTER 8

CIRCULATE YOUR QI: USING MOXA

Thousands of years ago, Chinese landowners would dig a hole on their property, fill it with dried mugwort leaf, and burn the leaves. After a while, steam would come up from the ground at various locations. The slow, intense heat of the burning mugwort, drawing on the Earth's energy meridians, had found water beneath the Earth's surface, indicating where the landowner should build a well.

Like Planet Earth, your body has energy meridians that reflect the Five Elements and connect with all the organs in your body. Women can follow the same wisdom used by ancient Chinese landowners to draw Qi to the acupuncture points that have a role in conception through a technique called *moxibustion*. In moxibustion, a dried herb called moxa—a form of mugwort—is burned near these points. When lit, moxa burns slowly and provides a penetrating heat and strong drawing power, which reinforces and activates Qi flow.

In my practice, I use moxibustion frequently. You may wish to obtain this treatment from a practitioner of Traditional Chinese Medicine, or you may opt to do it yourself—at your own risk. Please note that in certain states, buying or treating yourself with moxa is prohibited by law; to learn more, contact your local acupuncture board.

To use the technique described below, you'll need moxa sticks, which look a bit like large cigars. You can buy moxa sticks in Asian herb stores or online at a number of sites.

Note that if you seek treatment from a practitioner of Traditional Chinese

Medicine, he or she may use different forms of moxa to stimulate specific points to different degrees. We'll discuss these in Chapter 10.

HOW TO APPLY MOXA

To circulate your Qi in preparation for conception, take these steps at least once (and up to three times) per day. If you may be pregnant, morning and night are the best times to apply moxa.

1. Light the moxa stick by holding a match or lighter to either end and turning the stick slowly. Blow on it lightly, being careful not to scatter hot ashes. (It can take a bit of time to get the stick to burn evenly.) If you have trouble holding a match or lighter long enough to ignite your moxa, try this technique: Light a candle, then light your moxa stick from the candle's flame.

2. Identify the first acupuncture point you want to treat. (See pages 158–159 for a list of points recommended for the pre- and post-ovulation phases of your menstrual cycle.) Whichever sequence you follow, be sure to work from the top point to the bottom point (i.e., start with your head and end with your feet). If the point is on a limb, be sure to treat both sides of the body. (It doesn't matter whether you start on the left or the right.)

 BE CAREFUL!

If you choose to use moxa on yourself, be sure to exercise caution—you could burn yourself. Never touch your skin directly with the moxa stick, and be sure to flick off hot ashes frequently so they don't drop on your skin. Always perform moxibustion in a seated position rather than lying down. Be sure you've extinguished the stick completely after each use. And don't use moxa if you recently had major surgery, suddenly have developed a disease, or have a fever or infection.

WHAT'S THAT SMELL?

Moxa burns with a distinct, musky odor and can give off a lot of smoke. Some people find that the smell has a relaxing effect, while others find it difficult to tolerate. Smokeless stick moxa is available, but can be difficult to light; it also burns hotter, but with a subtle glow, so be careful not to hold the stick too close to your body. Experiment and see what works for you.

3. Before you apply the moxa, rub the point gently to wake up the Qi and alert your body that you are about to engage it in healing.

4. Hold the moxa stick about an inch above the point you are treating. To avoid overheating, move the moxa stick in a circular motion above the point; another technique is to move the stick repeatedly toward and away from the point. Do this for 2 to 5 minutes or until the point is comfortably warm, then move on to the next point. If you feel any discomfort, stop. The area should never become reddened from the heat. (If you're using the smokeless variety of moxa, be aware that it can be hotter than it appears; proceed with caution to avoid overheating the point or burning yourself.)

5. Once you've stimulated all the points in your sequence, extinguish your moxa stick, taking care that it does not continue to burn. The best way to extinguish a moxa stick is to deprive the embers of the oxygen they need to burn; you can achieve this by submerging the burning tip in a small jar of sand or rice, or by creating an aluminum-foil "cap" that will cover and extinguish the burning end of the stick. (Be careful not to hold the top of the cap, which can get hot and may burn your hand.) To prolong the life of your moxa stick, do not submerge it in water.*

6. After moxibustion, drink a small amount of warm water to help balance the warmth you've added to your body.

*You may think you've extinguished your moxa stick when you no longer see smoke, but please be cautious! The stick may remain hot even after the smoke disappears. Do not leave a recently extinguished moxa stick unattended.

MOXIBUSTION POINTS FOR WOMEN

Pre-Ovulation Moxibustion Points

Apply moxa daily to each of the points shown, depending on where you are in your menstrual cycle. Refer back to "How to Apply Moxa" on page 156 for instructions.

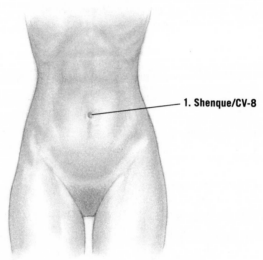

1. Shenque/CV-8

1. Location: Navel
   Corresponds to this acupuncture point: Shenque; Conception Vessel 8

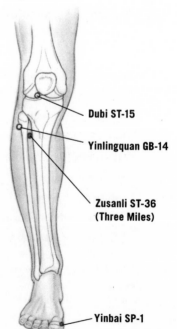

Dubi ST-15

Yinlingquan GB-14

Zusanli ST-36
(Three Miles)

Yinbai SP-1

2. Location: Just below the kneecap and slightly to the outside of the leg
   Corresponds to this acupuncture point: Zusanli Stomach 36

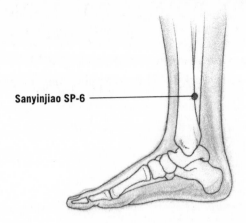

Sanyinjiao SP-6

3. Location: Inside of calf just above the ankle

   Corresponds to this acupuncture point: Sanyinjiao Spleen 6

POST-OVULATION

Note: If you become pregnant, continue using moxa on the post-ovulation points until week 28.

1. Location: Crown of the head

   Corresponds to this acupuncture point: Baihui Governing Vessel 20

2. Location: Just below the kneecap and slightly to the outside of the leg.

   Corresponds to this acupuncture point: Zuzanli Stomach 36

3. Location: Big toe at the bottom, outer corner of the toenail.

   Corresponds to this acupuncture point: Yinbai Spleen 1

Celia's Story
PATIENCE, PERSEVERANCE, AND AN EASTERN PERSPECTIVE

*B*etty conceived Stephen, her first child, using fertility drugs at age 42 and delivered him by C-section. Concerned that her biological clock was ticking, she and her husband started trying to conceive their second child when Betty stopped breastfeeding the first.

After 3 months of high-tech fertility cocktails, Betty still wasn't pregnant; her body seemed indifferent to the drugs. When she read an article in O *magazine questioning the safety of fertility drugs, she decided to give them up for good. She was not, however, willing to give up her hope for a second baby. Remembering something she'd read in the* San Francisco Chronicle *about a woman who was using Traditional Chinese Medicine to help infertile couples have miracle babies, she did an Internet search, found the article, and tracked me down.*

My examination showed Betty's constitution to be on the cool side, like that of the majority of women who come to our clinic. However, the temperature of her internal landscape was not Betty's only challenge. Her pale and purplish tongue revealed stagnation in her body. Sure enough, on Betty's abdomen was the scar from her previous C-section. Dark, rough, and tight compared to the rest of her skin, it indicated an incision that had healed in such a way that the flows of Blood and Qi to Betty's reproductive organs were hampered.

Improving the texture and color of Betty's scar became a focus of our work together. Betty used moxa to bring healing warmth to the scar, diligently applied ginger, and performed acupressure on the area. After about 2 months, she noticed that the scar had begun to change. But Betty realized it would take more time to bring her body fully into balance. Her question was: How much time? After 6 months of patient dedication to our Fertility Wisdom *program, she*

CLEARING A SCAR WITH GINGER MOXA

If your belly bears the scar of a previous C-section or surgery (even from child-hood), you can minimize the scar's impact on your future fertility by applying the dispersing properties of raw ginger and the healing warmth of moxa. Follow these steps two to three times per week:

1. Cut a slice of fresh ginger, making sure it contains a lot of juice.
2. With your fingertips, gently rub your scar three times in a clockwise direc-tion, then three times counterclockwise.
3. Gently rub the gingerroot on your scar so that the juice remains on your skin. (Do not leave the gingerroot itself on your skin.)
4. Light a moxa stick and, while it is warm but not too hot, move the moxa back and forth over the scar a few times. Be sure not to touch your skin.
5. After applying the moxa, rub the scar gently as in step 2 above.
6. As always when using moxa, drink a little warm water afterward.

began to wonder how much longer she should continue before giving up on pregnancy. In the 7th month, she conceived naturally, and 9 months later Celia was born—without a C-section.

CHAPTER 9

HARMONIZE YOUR ENVIRONMENT: FENG SHUI FOR FERTILITY

We've talked about harmonizing the Five Elements in your body through the foods you eat and the way you breathe. But you can also bring Wood, Fire, Earth, Metal, and Water into harmony by creating a beautiful and balanced environment around you.

Remember how Chinese pioneers used the herb mugwort to draw Water from the ground by tapping into the meridians of the planet? These same planetary meridians and the Qi that flows through them are available to us when we apply the ancient Chinese art of *feng shui*.

Feng shui puts Taoist concepts about energy and harmony in the natural world to work in the environments we create. Through the way we build on the land, place furniture and other objects in our homes, and choose colors for our décor and clothing, we can facilitate the flow of Qi around us and bring good fortune, health, harmony—even a baby—into our lives. Interior designers, architects, business moguls, movie stars, and everyday people planning their homes are using feng shui to help them achieve their goals. And you can, too—by putting a few basic principles into action, paying special attention to places in your house most associated with fertility, using color to harmonize your internal constitution, conjuring the power of ancient symbols, and, most important, taking a "whole house" approach to harmony.

FENG SHUI BASICS

Feng shui begins with the *Ba Gua,* pictured below.

Think of this mystical octagon as your blueprint for harmony. Each side of the Ba Gua represents a different aspect of life—Knowledge, Career, Wealth, Fame/Reputation, Relationships, Children, Helpful People, and Family. Each area is associated with one of the Five Elements and an organ of the body, as well as a color. By identifying which area of your home corresponds to which of the Ba Gua's aspects, you can take steps to ensure that your home's energies support your goal of conception.

The Ba Gua

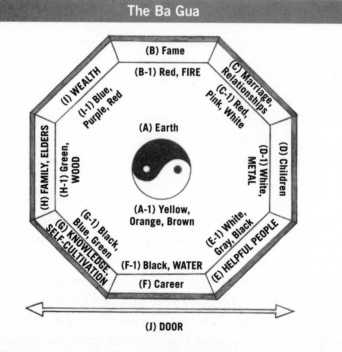

The Ba Gua is your blueprint for applying feng shui principles to your home, any room in it, or any environment where you spend time.

• **CENTER THE BA GUA** over your home or an individual room in your home • **ALIGN THE BOTTOM OF THE BA GUA** with the wall of your door • **YOUR DOOR WILL BE** in either the Knowledge (G), Career (F), or Helpful People (E) area on the Ba Gua • **SEE** which parts of your home/room correspond to different areas of your life

Start by tracing the Ba Gua in this book onto a piece of paper, indicating which side corresponds to Wealth, which to Relationships, and so on. Next, match the front door of your house to the side of the Ba Gua that corresponds with Career (the bottom of the diagram). Then sketch the outline of your house over the Ba Gua, indicating where the living room, bedrooms, bathroom, kitchen, and other rooms can be found. You now should have a map that tells you where to find the three aspects of your house most obviously related to fertility: Relationships, Children, and Family. These are the areas in which we will begin our work, putting several basic feng shui remedies in place.

Clear a path for Qi. Look around the rooms that represent Relationships, Children, and Family. Do the doors to these rooms open and close properly? Are the entrances blocked in any way? If so, make any changes necessary to allow Qi to enter and leave these rooms freely. Take the same steps with the front door to your house—the portal through which new Qi enters. Does a tree, a pole, or any other obstacle block the entrance? Or is there an open path for the energy of new life to come in?

Get rid of stagnation. Now assess these rooms for clutter. Are they full of unnecessary objects? Used for storage? Is there trash that needs to be taken out? Are closets or shelves neat and organized or in jam-packed disarray? Are there objects in these rooms that you can live without? Take steps now to make these rooms more vital and open by removing garbage, organizing storage spaces, and getting rid of objects you no longer use or need. (From a Taoist perspective, stagnant energy in your environment can reflect or lead to stagnant energy in your body.)

Circulate Qi. How long has it been since you gave these rooms a good cleaning, moved the furniture around, or reassessed your decorating scheme to create a pleasing environment? By moving, touching, and cleaning things in these rooms, you can get Qi moving and reacquaint yourself with the objects that surround you. Take a moment to appreciate the things that truly make you happy—and to consider a new future for things that don't.

Ensure safety and stability. Are there repairs to be made in these rooms that you've been putting off? Perhaps a leak in the roof? A window that

FENG SHUI TIPS

Feng shui puts Taoist concepts about energy and harmony in the natural world to work in the environments we create. To help create an environment conducive to health and fertility, follow these basic tips:

- To ensure balanced energy in your home, above the front door place one of the most basic tools of feng shui: a small mirror surrounded by the Ba Gua. Feng shui practitioners believe this symbol will protect your home and family—drawing in positive Qi and reflecting negative influences. (The Ba Gua mirror is a good energy remedy if the flow of Qi through your front door is impeded by a tree, lamppost, or other object.) Use this symbol to draw your attention to the presence of the Five Elements in your life by acknowledging and thanking it whenever you see it above your door. (You can find Ba Gua mirrors in many Asian markets, in feng shui specialty stores, or through a variety of sources online.)

- When placing furniture and other objects in your home or office, approach your task like an occupational therapist: Think "maximum benefit, minimum effort." Position things so you can reach them and use them easily, and so you can pass through rooms efficiently, without walking around furniture or piles of "stuff."

- Placing your bed according to feng shui principles can ensure restful sleep and a harmonious environment for conception. Position your bed so that, when you're in it, you can see the door but are not directly aligned with it. Avoid positioning the bed so that the foot of the bed points directly toward the door (symbolic of death), or the head is directly under a window (a position that can create insecurity in the sleeper).

- If your home's bathroom is in one of the sectors critical to conception (relationships, children, family), be sure there are no leaks in your plumbing, and keep the toilet seat down and the door closed—lest you lose vital fertility Qi down the drain!

- In your home, garden, office—any place where you spend a good deal of time—be sure that each of the Five Elements is represented by including all of their colors in your décor. For balance and harmony, you may also wish to include the full range of Five Element colors in your wardrobe.

won't open? An electrical outlet that doesn't work? Now is the time to make these repairs, turning your home into a place in which new life feels welcome and safe.

IN THE BEDROOM: REST AND ROMANCE

No matter which aspect of the Ba Gua it represents, your bedroom is an important place for peace and harmony when you're trying to conceive. Take a look at the room you sleep in. Is it clean and free of clutter? Dedicated to both peaceful slumber and procreation?

In the bedroom, it's particularly important that you not place unnecessary objects on the floor. (Is that a pile of dirty laundry in the corner? Are you storing winter clothing under your bed?) Clutter blocks the flow of Qi, and you want energy flowing freely in the room where you spend your sleeping life and likely will conceive your baby.

Ideally, your bedroom will be a place that supports rest and romance rather than distracting activities, so start by banning televisions, computers, exercise equipment, and other objects not dedicated to your primary bedroom objectives. Make this a place that reflects your commitment to conception, your clarity of purpose, and your enthusiasm for your ultimate goal.

THE POWER OF COLOR

As you may recall, each of the Five Elements corresponds to a different set of colors: green for Wood; red, pink, or orange for Fire; yellow, brown, or beige for Earth; white, gold, gray, or silver for Metal; and black, blue, or purple for Water. Color is a powerful feng shui remedy for restoring harmony; by using it in your external environment, you can bring balance and harmony to your internal landscape.

For example, you can balance a warmer constitution by being sure to

include cooling colors—white and blue, for Metal and Water—in your sur-
roundings. And you can warm a cooler constitution by conjuring Wood
and Fire through the color green, red, pink, or orange.

For simple fertility purposes, focus on bringing the warming or cooling
influence you need into your life by keeping the right colors close to you—
in the bedroom, where you spend so many hours of the night; and in the
clothes closest to your body, your underwear. In the interest of feng shui
fertility blessings, perhaps it's time for a change in color scheme: red, pink,
or orange underwear and/or sheets if your internal weather is cool; blue or
white if it's warm.

CALLING ON SYMBOLS

Feng shui masters know many remedies, both practical and esoteric, for
creating harmony in the home environment. Mirrors and crystals, living
plants, aquariums and fountains, bamboo flutes, the sound and motion
of bells and wind chimes, even electrical appliances—all can be used
to enliven or calm the Qi in a particular place in the interest of overall
harmony.

Some objects have symbolic value as feng shui remedies. By displaying
them in our homes, we tap into ancient beliefs and energies greater than
ourselves. The following symbols are considered auspicious for fertility. If
you choose to work with symbols, select those that have the most appeal
and meaning for you, and allow them to remind you of your goal whenever
you see them.

- Elephants: Elephants are associated with pregnancy. Placed on either
  side of the bedroom door, they are believed to enhance fertility.
- Dragons: A small statue or picture of a dragon can bring revitalizing
  Yang energy into your relationship when placed on the man's side of
  the bed.
- Red paper lanterns: Hung on either side of the bed, red lanterns are
  believed to have a Yang effect similar to a dragon statue.

• Fruit: Art depicting pomegranates, water chestnuts, lychees, longans, and lotus seeds is considered auspicious when fertility is desired.

A WHOLE-HOME APPROACH

Before you become overly focused on the rooms in your house with the most obvious connection to fertility, take a moment to consider that feng shui, like Traditional Chinese Medicine and the Taoist concepts that gave birth to both, is about wholeness. Just as we would not share the Inner Smile or the Healing Sounds with just one organ—or treat infertility in isolation from other aspects of health—the best feng shui approach focuses on your whole home, seeking harmony and balance across all aspects of life, from wealth to fame to family.

Think about it and you'll realize that all are equally critical to welcoming a baby into your life. A host of helpful people, there when you need them, is just as important as your primary relationship. And without reputation and knowledge, there may be no career, and without career, no wealth to support the child you seek to attract.

Once you've applied feng shui's Qi-enhancing initiatives to the parts of your home that represent relationships, children, and family, turn your newly aware eye to the rest of your home. Where else is there clutter you can clear out? Repairs you can make now? Beauty you can enhance?

One final note about feng shui: Those who discount it as superstition or hocus-pocus fail to recognize that a feng shui remedy, whether practical or symbolic, is just one step in a continuum that begins with intent (the inspiration that prompts us to consider a feng shui solution), takes shape through symbolic action (putting the feng shui remedy in place), and reverberates through the purposeful steps we then take to achieve our dreams. Believing a remedy will work is not enough. We must make that belief a constant in our lives and use it as the inspiration for ongoing action. Whenever we see a feng shui remedy at work—whether it's a fresh bedroom ceiling where a leak used to be, a well-organized linen closet, or a carved dragon by the bedside—we must bring our awareness back to our goal, thank the universe for its gifts, and, step by step, continue to move in the direction of our desired destination.

Christina's Story
FIVE ELEMENTS IN HARMONY

A few years ago, if you had asked Emma and Andy to name the Five Elements, they probably would have been able to guess at a few of them. But today, there is one element they will never forget; it's the missing link that brought them the baby it seemed nature would deny them.

Emma came to our clinic after trying to conceive for a year and a half without success and with the baffling Western diagnosis of unexplained infertility. Her menstrual cycle was as regular as clockwork, and she and Andy had no health complaints. But they were so frustrated with their inability to conceive that they were considering in vitro fertilization. Traditional Chinese Medicine, they hoped, would give them the edge toward the success that had long eluded them.

Checking the couple's internal weather, I saw no disharmonies that could not be overcome with gentle harmonizing and balancing through our Fertility Wisdom program. But looking at their birth dates and their Ba Zi charts—a window onto the Five Elements in their bodies and their lives—I saw something Emma and Andy would never have guessed: They both were missing the same element, Metal. If they continued to bring their bodies into harmony and balance, the cosmos would provide them with the Metal they needed when the season changed from late Summer to Fall, the season when Metal is at its energetic peak.

Skeptical yet hopeful, Emma and Andy let nature take its course. And as Summer gave way to Fall, with Metal at its peak, they conceived Christina, whose name will forever remind them of silver wind chimes, tinkling coins, and the wholeness that grows from Five Elements in harmony.

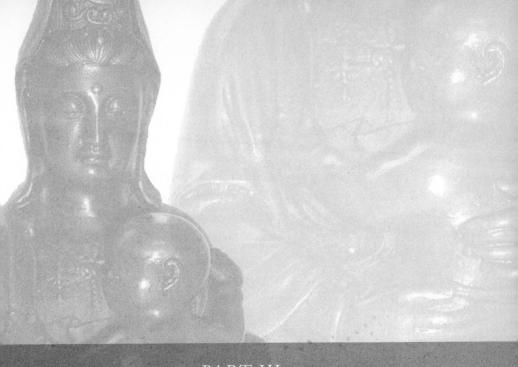

CULTIVATING PARTNERSHIPS

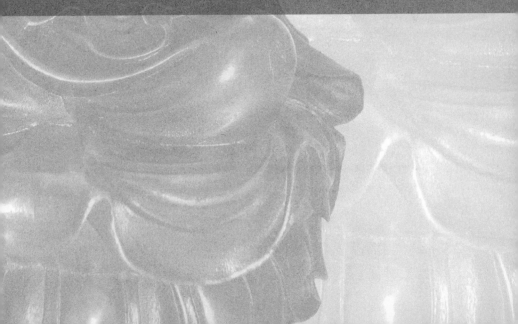

In my clinic, I advise my clients to give their bodies 3 to 6 months of preparation before attempting conception—then to try conceiving for another 3 to 6 months before assessing their progress. That means, realistically, you might follow our *Fertility Wisdom* program for as long as a year.

If, despite your best efforts, you've found yourself unable to welcome a baby into your life and you haven't yet sought the help of a practitioner of Traditional Chinese Medicine or a Western fertility expert, you owe it to yourself to take advantage of every available resource in order to achieve your goal. These resources include things you can do for yourself (like the practices outlined in this book) and helpful people (family, supportive friends, and health-care professionals) you can engage in your quest for a baby.

Our *Fertility Wisdom* empowers you to take profound steps toward fertility on your own, simply by aligning yourself with the laws of nature and by balancing and harmonizing your internal weather. However, I highly recommend that you undertake *Fertility Wisdom* with the support of a practitioner of Traditional Chinese Medicine, who can answer your questions, reinforce the energetic changes you're making in your body, and tailor this program to your constitution. You may also wish to work with a Western fertility expert—in which case you'll find *Fertility Wisdom* to be a good resource for managing the side effects of Western treatments. The pages that follow will help you forge productive relationships with both Eastern and Western health-care partners.

James's Story

TRAVELING AT THE SPEED OF PREGNANCY

Jennifer was running when she first came to our clinic. As one of the founders of a high-tech company, she rarely stopped thinking, hardly ever stood still, and frequently flew from one business destination to another. She'd been pregnant naturally seven times, had miscarried seven times, and had tried in vitro fertilization five

PARTNERING FOR SUCCESS

Working with health-care practitioners in order to conceive takes the same perspective and personal commitment required for any productive partnership:

- **Choose your partners carefully.** They should be professionals with whom you have a good rapport, whose perspective you understand and whose opinion you trust and respect, who answer questions to your satisfaction, who share your vision of how your pregnancy should unfold, and who demonstrate sincere caring for your welfare.
- **Be honest.** Have an open discussion with your professional partners about what you want and what you are and aren't willing to do to achieve your goal.
- **Take the initiative.** Ask questions and offer feedback. Raise difficult issues if they arise. And don't let an unanswered question turn into a lingering doubt or a growing fear.
- **Listen with an open mind.** Try to do this even if what you hear is strange, challenging, or discouraging. Then use good judgment to discern your own truth. And don't be afraid to seek a second or third opinion.
- **Be your own advocate.** When assessing what's right for you, call on your Three Treasures—Heaven (your reasoning brain), Human (your emotions), and Earth (your practical gut brain). Remember: In the end, only you are responsible for your success.
- **Be an ally—not an adversary.** Sometimes the challenges of understanding new health-care procedures and dealing with insurance and other administrative issues can make us feel at odds with the people who are trying to help us. Learn to smile and negotiate in the face of frustration.
- **Say thank you.** Gratitude is as good for the giver as it is for the receiver.

times without success. By the time Jennifer and I talked, doctors had already told her to consider donor eggs. She was running out of steam—and out of hope.

In our first meeting, Jennifer and I discussed how important it would be for her to change her lifestyle if she wanted to make room for a baby. We gave her a mantra: Slow down! We wrote it on her chart, and we repeated it to her frequently. We also gave her a new approach to eating and drinking—she and other clients she talked with called it the warm womb diet. Giving up favorite things was difficult, but she did it. And her husband became very good at cooking lamb and other dishes that would gently warm Jennifer's chilly internal landscape.

As she embraced this new, slower, warmer way of being, Jennifer found the hope she had lost in all her running, from meeting to meeting, fertility specialist to IVF procedure. She conceived naturally at age 46 and, 9 months later, brought James into a Western world that once regarded him as an impossible dream.

CHAPTER 10

WORKING WITH A PRACTITIONER OF TRADITIONAL CHINESE MEDICINE

All of the stories in this book are based on the experiences of real people who brought home their babies by using aspects of our *Fertility Wisdom* on their own. They changed their eating and drinking habits to harmonize their internal weather. They practiced the meditation techniques and Qi Gong exercises you've just learned. They drew upon the healing energy of their own hands and learned to use acupressure on themselves. They also visited our clinic for treatments—the same internal organ acupressure techniques outlined in this book, the same moxa applications you've learned to perform on yourself, plus acupuncture treatments, which further balanced and harmonized their constitutions, and "cupping"—an age-old practice that gets Qi circulating and helps rid the body of toxins.

If you seek treatment from a practitioner of Traditional Chinese Medicine, the techniques recommended in this book can support your Eastern practitioner's efforts to bring balance, harmony, and congruency to your body.

WELCOME TO A NEW WORLD OF HEALING

When you enter the offices of a practitioner of Traditional Chinese Medicine, you walk into a world informed by a centuries-old system of beliefs and prac-

LOOKING FOR A PRACTITIONER OF TRADITIONAL CHINESE MEDICINE?

Trying to find an Eastern practitioner—particularly one who specializes in fertility—but not sure where to start? Here are some suggestions:

- Ask friends, relatives, and those in the medical community for suggestions. If you're working with a Western fertility specialist, perhaps he or she has other clients who are combining Western and Eastern approaches to fertility and can recommend a practitioner of Traditional Chinese Medicine.
- Ask for suggestions from alternative medical practitioners, such as chiropractors, massage therapists, homeopaths and naturopaths.
- Research local practitioners of Traditional Chinese Medicine on the Internet, looking for those with a specialty in fertility.
- Check out your health plan's Web site, which may list qualified, covered practitioners.

Once you have identified some practitioners to choose from, make appointments and interview them to ensure that you find the best partner for you. Before the interviews, make a list of the top characteristics you believe a practitioner should have—for example, knowledge, experience, warmth, competence, honesty, accessibility, promptness, friendliness, professionalism, good listening skills, compatibility, and communication skills. Keep these characteristics in mind as you interview potential practitioners.

Here are some questions you may wish to ask during your interviews:

- What are your qualifications and training? (Acupuncturists must be certified by their state or national board.) How long have you practiced Traditional Chinese Medicine?
- What is your approach to fertility treatment?
- What experiences and results have you had with fertility treatment?
- Are you comfortable with my seeing both you and a Western doctor for fertility treatment? Are you willing to adapt your treatments, if necessary, to support my Western doctor's efforts (for example, supporting hormonal stimulation or suppression)?
- How do you feel about clients who ask a lot of questions?
- Will you be accessible if I call with a question between treatments?
- Can you provide testimonials from other fertility clients, or do you have fertility clients who would be willing to discuss their experiences with me?

tices—a world that is very different from the Western approach to medicine.

If this is your first treatment with Traditional Chinese Medicine, you undoubtedly have many questions about what to expect. And even if you've been seeing an Eastern practitioner for a while, you may still wonder about certain aspects of your treatment. The information that follows will help you understand what you experience when you visit a practitioner of Traditional Chinese Medicine and help you make the most of your partnership.

BEFORE YOUR VISIT

Our *Fertility Wisdom* guidelines ask you to abstain from alcohol, coffee, smoking, and drugs (except prescribed medications) while you are attempting to conceive and throughout your pregnancy. This advice also applies to the 24 hours before you visit a practitioner of Traditional Chinese Medicine. These substances can cause symptoms that could be misinterpreted by your practitioner—and may also disrupt the effects of your treatment.

Keep in mind that clinical studies have shown that your stomach should be neither empty nor full before an acupuncture treatment. Having an empty stomach during treatment might cause you to feel dizzy, nauseous, or even faint, while you may become nauseous or even vomit if you are too full. If it's been a long time since you've eaten, have a light snack before your appointment.

INTAKE AND ASSESSMENT

In order to determine how to bring your body into harmony and balance, your Eastern practitioner will use five traditional methods of diagnosis (as I mentioned in Chapter 2). Some of these techniques will be familiar to you from your Western experience. For example, your practitioner may ask for a detailed medical history when you visit for the first time. Be sure to bring information related to your attempts to conceive, including the results of any hormone-level (FSH/LH) tests for you and any sperm analysis for your partner, taken within the past 3 months. I consult these results in my practice, and your practitioner may, as well.

Like a Western doctor, your Eastern practitioner will ask direct questions about your health. However, some of your Eastern practitioner's questions may not seem to apply to your desire to conceive—at least not from a Western perspective. For example, in addition to questions about your menstrual patterns, you may be asked about your overall energy level, bowel movements, frequency of urination, sensations of heat or cold throughout your body, sensations of thirst, sleep patterns, and emotional state.

Remember that Traditional Chinese Medicine treats the whole person—body, mind, and spirit. To help you attract new life, your practitioner must assess health patterns that reflect the way energy flows through your body. Because all of our organs act in concert, a complaint in one area may reflect an imbalance that originates in a seemingly unrelated organ. Also, things like sleep, thirst, and bowel movements tell a lot about your general energy, constitution, and ability to digest food and eliminate toxins.

In addition to asking questions, your practitioner will use other methods of investigation: observing your appearance and behavior, examining your tongue, noting the smell of your breath and body, listening to the tone of your voice and the sound of your breathing and coughing, and touching you to determine how cool or warm and dry or damp you are—and to feel your pulses.

Based on all of these methods of investigation, your practitioner will determine how best to stimulate, clear, and/or redirect your body's energy to balance and harmonize your internal weather—and increase your chances of conceiving.

PREPARATORY TREATMENT

To prepare your body for acupuncture, your practitioner may perform one or more of a variety of techniques:

ACUPRESSURE

Acupressure is the use of massage techniques and meridian stretches to redirect Qi along the body's meridians. These techniques can also help your practitioner to determine the condition of your meridians and diagnose which meridians are related to any physical complaints you may have.

HOW YOU CAN HELP

At each appointment, your Eastern practitioner will ask questions about your health. To make the most of your treatments, monitor your body on an ongoing basis and come to your visits prepared to provide information on these aspects of your health.

- **Your menstrual cycle:** Are your periods regular? How long do they typically last? How would you describe your menstrual flow: Is it bright red? Clotted? When do you ovulate? Designating the first day of your menstrual cycle as Day 1, what day is it in your cycle?
- **Your bowel movements:** Do you move your bowels every day? Are your bowel movements usually constipated or loose? Do you have bouts of diarrhea or constipation? If so, do you have them irregularly, in response to what you eat, or at particular times of your cycle? Do you have blood in your stool? Is your stool unusually pale or dark? Are you passing any undigested food?
- **Sensations of heat and cold in your body:** Do you have cold hands and/or feet? Are you frequently thirsty? Do you notice sensations of heat anywhere in your body?
- **Sleep patterns:** Do you have trouble falling asleep? Do you wake up during the night? How frequently and at what times? Can you get back to sleep? What is your energy level when you wake up—are you ready to get up and go, or not?
- **General energy level:** Are you tired or energetic at particular times of the day? In certain weather or certain seasons?
- **Emotional state:** Do you feel particularly angry, sad, worried, anxious, or happy? Do you notice stress-related symptoms in your body, such as stomach discomfort, muscle tension, or headaches? Do these symptoms change based on what you eat, how well you sleep, or how hard you are working? Do they change based on where you are in your menstrual cycle?

If you are also seeing a Western fertility expert, be prepared to tell your Eastern practitioner what protocol your Western expert is using and where you are in that cycle. For example: Are you taking hormones? Getting ready for egg retrieval? Preparing for implantation? Your Eastern practitioner may be able to adapt his or her treatment strategy to support your Western treatments.

CUPPING

Cupping is an ancient technique used to stimulate and clear Qi and Blood along the same meridians used in acupuncture and acupressure. The practitioner uses a flame to create a vacuum inside a heavy glass dome, or "cup," then applies the cup to your back and other areas. The cup adheres to the skin through suction, drawing blood to the body's external capillaries.

Your practitioner may apply three or four cups at a time—or more when necessary. He or she may allow the cups to simply rest on specific acupuncture points or move them along the body for a few minutes. Occasionally the suction created by the cups will leave mild redness or marking that usually disappears within 24 to 72 hours.

Cupping is particularly effective in improving circulation, clearing cold or flu congestion, and treating other conditions characterized by stagnation.

MOXIBUSTION

In chapter 8, we discussed how you can facilitate the flow of Qi to certain acupuncture points through moxibustion. Your Traditional Chinese Medicine practitioner may use stick moxa to stimulate certain points, or burn loose moxa on a fresh slice of ginger or a mixture of garlic, salt, and herbs, then apply it to your skin. Or, after acupuncture needles are inserted, your practitioner may form loose moxa into cones, place them on the needles, and light them.

ACUPUNCTURE

Acupuncture is perhaps the most familiar element among the practices we know as Traditional Chinese Medicine; some practitioners specialize in acupuncture alone, without offering cupping, herbs, or other traditional treatments.

Acupuncture is the insertion of thin, sterile needles of various sizes along the body's energy channels, or meridians (including the ear), to stimulate, clear, or redirect body energy (Qi). When your practitioner inserts needles along these meridians, neural signals are released that can have a variety of effects on your body, including inhibiting pain, eliminating muscle tension, improving bloodflow, promoting tissue healing, strengthening your immune response, and restoring the functional balance of internal organs.

After assessing your condition by asking you questions, examining you, and feeling your pulses—and perhaps after preparing your body with acupressure, cupping, and/or moxibustion—your practitioner will insert needles in a pattern designed to rebalance your energy for optimal health. Typically you will lie on your back or stomach during the treatment. It takes just a few seconds to insert each needle. Then you'll be asked to rest with the needles in place for a period of time that is determined by your condition. During that time, it's important to relax and remain still, breathing in and appreciating your body.

 ## HOW DOES ACUPUNCTURE FEEL?

Everyone's response to needles is different, and one person's response can vary from visit to visit depending on general health and where the needle is being placed on the body. Some people report no sensation whatsoever when needles are inserted. Others describe the treatment as feeling like a mosquito bite, and still others say they feel a heavy sensation or what seems like a brief electrical shock. However, many say that the overall feeling of relaxation that occurs once the needles are inserted is well worth any temporary discomfort.

If you are anxious about having acupuncture needles inserted, tell your practitioner. He or she may recommend breathing or other techniques to help you receive needles without discomfort.

If you feel discomfort while the needles are in place, tell your practitioner right away. To help you relax and bring your awareness back to your physical body, breathe to the place you feel pain, imagining that each inhalation is bringing healing energy to the point, and that each exhalation is clearing out discomfort.

When needles are in place, some people also experience profound emotions that may or may not reflect their feelings when they arrived for their treatment. In Chinese medical theory, each organ is associated with a set of emotions or virtues—for example, sadness/bravery for the lungs, fear/calmness for the kidneys. These emotions may be triggered and released when needles stimulate related acupuncture points. If you feel strong emotions, ask your practitioner for assistance. Also, keep in mind that this simply means your body is clearing long-term blockages that may have limited your chances of conceiving.

FOLLOWING TREATMENT

After you have rested with the needles in place, your practitioner will remove them. Take a moment to relax before you get up. After treatment, I suggest you drink some warm water to help your body maximize the benefits of your treatment.

Your Eastern practitioner may prescribe Chinese herbs to support your acupuncture treatments. Prescriptions may take the form of a premade liquid, powder, pill, or capsule, or you may be prescribed dried herbs that you cook at home. Some of the herbal remedies traditionally used to address infertility are standardized, patented formulas. You'll find information on these formulas in Appendix E on page 221. *Note: Please do not take these formulas or any other herbal remedies without the guidance of a practitioner of Traditional Chinese Medicine.*

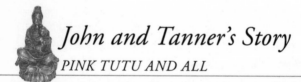

John and Tanner's Story
PINK TUTU AND ALL

*E*verything went well with Lila's first pregnancy until the 37th week, when an umbilical cord abnormality took the life of the boy she would have delivered 3 weeks later. By the time she and her husband, Frank, decided to try again, Lila was 38. Although she'd gotten pregnant right away when she was younger, her doctor told her not to expect fast results this time. Because of her age, he said, Lila should try any and every means possible to improve her chances of conception.

Lila and Frank started with a top fertility expert, who told them Lila's uterine lining was too thin; they might as well start looking for a surrogate to carry their baby, he said. Not ready to accept that recommendation, they consulted another leading fertility expert. With Lila's FSH at 18, that specialist said he felt it would be unethical to take their money and try to treat Lila—her chances of con-

ceiving were that slim. Still not willing to give up, they begged the doctor to take them on, and he agreed to try.

Looking for every advantage, Lila had already been coming to our clinic for 2 months when she began work with the second fertility expert. It came as no surprise to Lila when I informed her that she would have to warm her cooler constitution; she had already noticed that she felt chilly most of the time, and that her energy was low. (In fact, an endocrinologist had diagnosed her as having an underactive thyroid gland.)

To balance and harmonize her cooler constitution, Lila had been making dramatic changes in what she ate and drank. She had also been using moxa diligently to warm key pregnancy points. Anything I asked of her, she would do, Lila said, if it would increase her chances of a healthy pregnancy. ("If you asked me to wear a pink tutu and walk up and down Clement Street on my hands, I'd do it," she once said.)

Her commitment was paying off: Her body was beginning to warm up; she had more energy. At the same time, she diligently followed the advice of her Western fertility doctor, keeping our clinic informed of the procedures she was undergoing so we could support Western methods with Eastern techniques.

Her Western doctor remained skeptical, but at each step Lila turned his expectations upside down: When he didn't think she would produce enough follicles, she produced 10. When he doubted that any would produce viable embryos, 10 were fertilized. When he warned Lila and Frank that not all of the embryos would survive, all of them lived the 3 days between fertilization and transfer. But when the time came for transfer, tests showed that Lila's uterine lining was still too thin. Disappointed but dedicated, Lila agreed to have the embryos frozen and to take a month off to allow her body to recover from the hormone bombardment of pre-IVF treatments. And it was in that month off that Lila got pregnant—naturally. Nine months later, John was born.

Eager to take advantage of what they knew would be a shrinking opportunity to enlarge their family, Lila and Frank nurtured John and, when he was old enough to be weaned, rededicated themselves to harmonizing Lila's body through Eastern medicine. Then they went back to their Western fertility expert for a consultation about conceiving again. Little did they know, as they sat in the doctor's office, that Lila, 42 years old, was already pregnant with Tanner, born happy and healthy 9 months later—and Lila didn't even have to wear a tutu.

CHAPTER 11

WORKING WITH A WESTERN FERTILITY EXPERT

In my practice I frequently share clients with Western fertility experts. Sometimes it's the clients who bring awareness of Traditional Chinese Medicine to their Western doctors. And often Western doctors who are familiar with my practice refer clients they think will benefit from blending Western and Eastern approaches.

If you plan to use our *Fertility Wisdom* in conjunction with Western treatments—or if you plan to consult with both Western and Eastern specialists while following this program—there are a few things you should know.

A WORD ABOUT HERBS

By now, many Western fertility experts are familiar with acupuncture and are aware of research conducted by the National Institutes of Health demonstrating that acupuncture can enhance the effectiveness of Western fertility strategies. If you are pursuing Western fertility treatment, be sure to tell your doctor that you are also following a self-care program based on the same concepts as acupuncture: a gentle and noninvasive approach combining nutrition, exercise, acupressure, and meditation to prepare the body for pregnancy—one that in no way interferes with Western treatments.

In particular, your Western doctor will want to know if you are taking any herbal remedies. Even Western fertility specialists who recommend acupuncture to their clients may be wary of herbs, for two good reasons.

First, in order for Western Assisted Reproductive Technologies to work, your specialist must be able to predict and control your hormones, stimulating or suppressing them for a desired effect at particular times. Your Western doctor may be concerned that herbs will have an unmanageable effect on your body's production of hormones, altering your response to Western procedures in unpredictable ways.

Second, Western fertility doctors may be concerned about the quality and safety of herbal treatments. It's true that herbs are powerful remedies—some are dangerous—and many people don't understand how to use them properly. So please, don't self-prescribe herbal remedies you've heard might enhance fertility. It takes knowledge and expertise to concoct and select safe and appropriate herbal formulas, and you and your potential baby are too precious to risk.

If you're working with a practitioner of Traditional Chinese Medicine who has prescribed herbs for you, be aware that your Western fertility expert may ask you not to take these formulas, even if he or she does not understand what they are. Of course, the decision is up to you, but whatever you decide—to take the herbs or not to take the herbs—be at peace with your choice. If you choose not to take the herbs, tell your Eastern practitioner so that he or she can adjust your treatments accordingly. And if you choose to take herbs, take the initiative to educate your Western doctor about their impact. Research the effects of each herb in any formula and share that information with your Western doctor.

(In our clinic, herbs play an important role in our work to balance and harmonize bodies prior to pregnancy. I personally developed the formulas we prescribe, based on my long experience with herbs and with fertility clients. In addition, a company that has earned my respect and patronage through many years of working together manufactures these formulas; I feel confident that these formulas are produced according to the highest quality and safety standards. However, sometimes a client will have reservations about taking herbs because his or her Western doctor has recommended against it. In these situations, my client's comfort is my ultimate goal; if taking the herbs creates stress and conflict, I will continue to work with the client, using other Eastern tools to compensate.

RELIEF FROM SIDE EFFECTS

If you've tried Western Assisted Reproductive Technologies before, you know they can have a powerful and not always positive impact, both physically and emotionally. On high dosages of potent fertility drugs, many women experience severe bloating, to the point where even their tongues swell. What's more, these women may feel emotionally out of control, with extreme highs and lows, or angry and aggressive.

Women following our *Fertility Wisdom* in conjunction with Western treatments rarely experience these side effects. And if they do, they have tools at their disposal to help them bring their bodies into better balance and harmony. If you find yourself feeling bloated and emotional, spend more time opening your Wind Gates, as described on page 106. Transform destructive emotions into supportive emotions by doing the Laughing Qi Gong exercise on page 135 and the Six Healing Sounds on page 123. And bring your whole body into greater harmony by spending extra time on the Inner Smile meditation described on page 117.

PROTECTING AFTER TRANSFER

If you're undergoing in vitro fertilization, take extra precautions with your precious potential cargo after the transfer of embryos to your body. As you

AFTER WESTERN FERTILITY TREATMENTS— A SIMPLE DETOX

If you've tried Western fertility intervention without success, you already know the toll fertility drugs and procedures can take on your body. If you are adopting our Eastern approach after ongoing Western treatments, the best thing you can do for your body is to cleanse it of toxins and residual fertility drugs before proceeding. (If you're continuing with Western treatments, you can also do a simple detox before beginning another cycle of Western fertility treatments). Here's how:

- **Intensify efforts to avoid foods on your "Don't!" list.** Our *Eating and Drinking Wisdom* asks you to avoid sugar, wheat, dairy, coffee, alcohol, processed foods with additives and preservatives, and high-fat foods. If you've been slipping from these guidelines, now is the time to embrace them with renewed vigor.

- **Avoid foods known to cause allergic reactions—even if you don't think you're allergic to them.** Eliminate corn and corn products, yeast, and sources of gluten (found in many grains, including wheat, barley, oats, rye, spelt, and kamut).

- **Drink plenty of room- or body-temperature water.** Proper hydration is essential to eliminating waste from the body. Don't let yourself go thirsty—drink *before* you become thirsty. And make sure you're drinking enough fluids every day. If you drink fruit juices, dilute them with water by half.

- **Chew thoroughly.** Remember, digestion begins in the mouth.

- **Choose proteins carefully.** Eat a little beef or fish (except tuna, swordfish, shark, and other mercury-heavy fish), but avoid lamb, poultry, and shellfish.

- **Improve bowel function.** Regular, healthy bowel movements—every day, and neither too loose nor too firm—are critical to helping your body cleanse itself of toxins. To generate a good bowel movement, be sure your meals include lots of cooked leafy greens and, unless your constitution is cooler, fruits—except citrus (especially grapefruit, which contains a compound that inhibits production of liver-cleansing enzymes), melon, mango, and pineapple.

- **Drink green tea.** Rich in antioxidants and slightly cooling, it's a good remedy for clearing toxins and stagnation.

- **Take a detox bath.** In a tub of warm (not hot) water, dissolve 1 cup of sea salt and 1 cup of baking soda. Step in and relax!

would after ovulation if there's a chance you're pregnant, avoid travel, intense exercise, and emotionally stimulating situations. And refrain from all acupressure or massage below the navel and on the shoulders. (Remember, massaging the shoulders can stimulate acupuncture points that encourage energy to move down in the body. That means no shoulder rubs, Uterine Lift or Groin Pulse Acupressure, and Wind Gates no lower than three o'clock and nine o'clock.

DIFFERENT PERSPECTIVES, SHARED GOALS

As you proceed in your efforts to conceive, perhaps engaging the support of Eastern and Western professional partners, keep this in mind. Although they may hold dramatically different perspectives on fertility and use different tools to enhance it, Western and Eastern health-care professionals have one thing in common: They want you to succeed. They want you to have the baby you so desire.

Perhaps, like some of the women I see in our clinic, you've had difficult experiences with Western fertility treatments in the past—failed in vitro fertilization, miscarriages after hard-won pregnancies, doctors who deliver disheartening diagnoses or tell you your chances of conceiving are next to none. Maybe you've even tried acupuncture or other alternative health approaches without success.

It's time now to put those experiences behind you. Acknowledge the good intentions of the people who tried to help you in the past, even if their efforts disappointed or discouraged you. Let go of any guilt, fear, or self-doubt left over from previous fruitless attempts at pregnancy; replace those feelings with a positive outlook by—yes—smiling to and thanking your body for its efforts. Remember, conception is the baby's choice, not a product of your will or your professional partner's skill. And you can improve your chances of being that choice by nurturing, encouraging, and supporting the best partner you have: your body.

Laura and Amanda's Story
GIVE YOUR BODY A SECOND CHANCE

*J*essica looked forward to the day she would bring her first baby home; she cherished the thought of those first months of bonding. But when she went into the hospital to give birth, things went terribly wrong. A torn placenta during delivery left Jessica badly hemorrhaging, and her doctor had to reach inside her to manually reposition her distressed uterus. Having forgone any form of anesthesia in favor of natural childbirth, Jessica says it was the most painful thing she's ever experienced.

This traumatic event haunted Jessica in spirit and body. Home with her new daughter, Laura, she began to experience extreme anxiety and felt even more fatigued than she had expected. Her thyroid went haywire—underactive, then normal, then underactive again. Then, 14 months after delivering Laura, Jessica got her period again, but found she'd lost something else: her sense of smell. Jessica felt sicker and more isolated than she'd ever been in her life.

Eventually Jessica and her husband decided to add to their family while they were still fertile. But after 6 months of trying— including a few miscarriages—Jessica, 42, still wasn't pregnant. With her trust in medicine damaged after her first childbirth experience, Jessica sought an alternative: She came to our clinic. Little did she know, as she sat in our waiting room, that she was already pregnant.

Jessica's health history and her extremely overheated and dry constitution—evident in her bright red tongue and high anxiety—told me that, to ensure a healthy pregnancy, we would have to cool and balance her internal weather and strengthen key organs, including her lungs, which govern the immune system and can carry old feelings of sadness. During one treatment, Jessica began to weep uncontrollably. She continued to sob for a half hour after leaving the clinic, she later told me.

Meditating on the incident, Jessica came to realize she was releasing old grief—for the loss of her health, the loss of her trust in medicine, and the lost dream of those first blissful months at home with Laura. It was a breakthrough moment, physically and emotionally, in our work to bring Jessica back to life, even as she carried new life inside her.

Since that time, Jessica has given birth to Amanda—an easy birth, particularly compared to her first experience. She's navigated other challenges and losses—the death of her mother, Laura's medical problems—without compromising her health. The anxiety she had felt since Laura was born has diminished. And slowly but surely, her sense of smell is returning. As Jessica continues to work with me and to heal herself, she's beginning to notice a truth she had long forgotten: That the world into which she was reborn, along with Amanda, is full of promise, and fragrant with flowers.

EPILOGUE

BLESSINGS BEYOND BABIES

In this journey we call life, each of us travels in a different vehicle. The vehicle we drive—the body we inhabit—is determined by our spirit's choice at the moment we are conceived.

Some of us choose sports cars—sleek, built for speed, perhaps a little temperamental and pricey to maintain. Others choose practical models—a reliable, low-maintenance truck or station wagon, or maybe an energy-efficient hybrid sedan. Still others among us choose to make our way in jalopies. As we travel along, it seems like we're stopping every half-mile to patch a tire, fill the radiator, or replace the fan belt.

Although we cannot swap the body that is our destiny for a different model, we *do* make choices throughout our lives that determine the path we follow and the quality of the road beneath us—winding or straight, bumpy or smooth. And at every fork in the road, at every turn, we have a fresh opportunity to change course.

I offer this analogy because, often, the men and women I meet in my practice come in discouraged by bodies that have failed to produce babies, or blaming life choices that seem to put them at the wrong time and place for pregnancy ("Why did I put off childbearing to have a career?" "Why didn't I take better care of myself in my twenties?").

Now, as you prepare your body to welcome a baby spirit whose arrival you cannot control, is the time to make peace with your own choices—the one your spirit made before you were born, and those you have made since.

Perhaps your spirit chose a vehicle whose capabilities do not match the journey you now envision for yourself. Perhaps the path you've followed in life places you off course for your desired destination. As you consider what you'd like to achieve and experience in life, keep in mind that although you cannot change vehicles mid-journey or change the direction in which you've already come, from this point forward, you can choose the road you travel. You can choose to turn right or left at the next signpost. You can choose the bumpy dirt back road or the meandering scenic route, the paved superhighway or cross-town streets. You can improve your journey by fueling and maintaining your vehicle with loving care. And whatever the condition of your vehicle and the direction of your path, you can choose to travel with an open mind and a smile on your face.

WHEN YOU BECOME PREGNANT

If our traditional Chinese wisdom helps you welcome the baby you desire, please accept my congratulations and blessings! Now, I have just one favor to ask of you: Please respect and protect the precious seed within you.

In my many years of helping infertile couples conceive, I have had plenty of opportunity to ponder the philosophical implications of my role in uniting hopeful parents with miracle babies they might not have welcomed otherwise. It's a responsibility I do not take lightly.

As an ambassador for Quan Yin and her generous gift of fertility, I also consider myself a spokesperson for baby spirits—someone who must communicate honestly with potential parents. If the tiny seed inside you could speak, it would say: "Please see the world as I do. I am small—not even as big as a pea—and I am so vulnerable!" If you conceive, I ask you to heed that little voice before saying to yourself: "At last, I'm pregnant! Now I can get on with my life!"

Before you abandon our *Eating and Drinking Wisdom* and celebrate with a piece of chocolate cake, before you run to the gym for a prenatal yoga class, before you hop on a plane to share the happy news in person with your parents, before you leap out of bed in the morning without doing the Inner Smile meditation, before you cancel your next appointment with your acupuncturist because it's just too expensive, and, besides, you've achieved your goal—remember the lessons you learned in the garden, about maintaining harmony and nurturing the foundation for new life. Before you celebrate the results of your ultrasound, thinking the hard part is over, consider that maintaining the harmony and balance you've established will be critical to a full-term healthy pregnancy. Before you jump and jostle and stress the little seed inside and feed toxins into the soil that supports it, remember that you are not quite the same person who first set out in search of fertility. You are carrying a precious passenger, and your true journey has just begun.

For many formerly infertile couples, the real challenges start after they deliver their baby. Depleted from 9 months of pregnancy and the challenges of childbirth, some new mothers feel overwhelmed, depressed, even suicidal. Here they are, blessed with the baby they've wanted for so long—a baby whose only voice is an insistent cry—and they can barely muster the physical and emotional strength to care for their new arrival.

Now is not the time to abandon the healthful practices that have brought you this far. In fact, it's time to return to your practitioner of Traditional Chinese Medicine (if you've consulted one) for an updated diagnosis, since pregnancy and childbirth can affect your constitution. (I recommend that

---

 FIRST TRIMESTER REMINDER

So many pregnancies end in miscarriage during the first trimester because newly pregnant mothers fail to recognize the fragility of their new passenger. We've discussed this before, but as a humble spokesperson for future babies, I cannot remind you enough of the following precautions. During the first trimester of pregnancy, or if you think you might be pregnant:

- Avoid travel by air or by car on bumpy roads.
- Get gentle, upper-body exercise only—nothing vigorous.
- Abstain from sexual rigorous activity.
- Replace baths with short, warm showers, and avoid swimming.
- Avoid intense emotional experiences.
- Stay away from spicy foods.
- No shoulder rubs.
- Do not use scented products such as bath oils, essential oils, incense, candles, sachets, lotions, and perfumes.
- Avoid ginger juice and dried ginger.

mothers return to my clinic no later than three months after delivery.) Your baby needs you to be strong, to be a source of nourishment as you've been for 9 months. New mothers who stick to our *Fertility Wisdom*—continuing to eat and drink for internal harmony, continuing to find time for the Six Healing Sounds and other practices—find they have more energy to care for their babies, higher-quality milk, and a better attitude about the challenges ahead. And women who take the time to heal themselves after pregnancy—performing the Uterine Lift and Groin Pulse Acupressure regularly, continuing to rely on herbs and acupuncture if these tools were part of their pre-pregnancy regimen—find that their general health improves quickly, their pelvic muscles regain their fitness, they enjoy sex sooner (so important for reconnecting with their partner in parenting), and they're better prepared for their next pregnancy, if they choose to invite another child into the family.

WHEN YOU DO NOT BECOME PREGNANT

In China, where acupuncture and other Eastern treatments are readily available and inexpensive compared to their costs in the West, fertility is not considered a specialty in Traditional Chinese Medicine or a last-ditch luxury for hopeful parents. It's just another part of whole-body health.

Many couples who come to our clinic understand why. Whether or not they conceive, they often feel as though they are in better general health. Digestive problems and allergies disappear. Complexions improve. Aches and pains diminish. Stamina increases and concentration improves. They simply feel better equipped to handle life's challenges—even if one of those challenges is accepting the fact that they have not yet welcomed a baby.

If you have followed all aspects of our *Fertility Wisdom* program for 3 to 6 months and you still have not conceived, it's time to pause for reevaluation. Have you tried all aspects of the program—from the *Eating and Drinking Wisdom* to the Qi Gong exercises—with 100 percent dedication? (Remember our talk about becoming 75 percent pregnant in exchange for a 75 percent commitment? It just doesn't add up that way.) Have you consulted with a Western fertility expert to see if there are special circumstances preventing your pregnancy? (For example, Western technology, in conjunction with Eastern wisdom for the sake of good health, offers the best hope for women whose Fallopian tubes are completely blocked.) Have both members of your partnership—male and female—been checked for overall health and reproductive wellness? (Remember our story about the young woman who worked tirelessly to harmonize her internal garden while her husband insisted his sperm wasn't the issue? As it turned out, he had virtually no seed to plant.) Have you considered boosting your chances by using this program in conjunction with acupuncture treatments, or by trying Western and Eastern approaches in sync?

If you answered "yes" to all of these questions and still have not conceived, I ask you to look, once again, deeper within, to your true feelings about having a baby. Are your Three Treasures—head, heart, and gut— truly in alignment? Is real desire, unmitigated by fear, guilt, or doubt, truly powering your efforts—or might old feelings be blocking your access to the one resource every infertile couple needs: hope? (How many clients have I seen get pregnant when they're taking a break from Western high-tech treatments and no longer thinking of their success or failure at conception? How many have made an appointment weeks in advance, come in for a consultation full of new hope, and later found they were already pregnant before even showing me their tongues?)

Finally, I ask you to broaden your perspective and recognize that life can bring us blessings—and opportunities to celebrate new life—well beyond babies. The philosophy, tools, and techniques in this book are not just a good way to get pregnant. They're a pathway to miracles we may not even recognize when we set our sites exclusively on conception.

FERTILITY WISDOM EQUALS LIFE WISDOM

If you have tried the tools in this book and found any that simply make you feel better, I hope you will make them part of your everyday life. Understanding the concept of internal weather, listening to your body, recognizing how your constitution can change with seasons and circumstances—warmer some days, cooler others—can be the first step to a lifetime of good health.

For women, the same organs that support conception and pregnancy are critical to whole-body health, whether you're a young woman just beginning her menstrual cycles or a mature woman approaching or beyond menopause. By eating and drinking for balance and harmony; by aligning body, mind, and spirit through simple practices like Opening the Wind Gates and the Inner Smile; and by keeping Qi circulating in your body and in your environment, you can maintain healthy menstrual cycles and navigate transitions in your reproductive life in comfort. So if it works for you, use it—if not for pregnancy, then for the rest of your life.

We call it *Fertility Wisdom,* the gift of Quan Yin. But in its approach to fertility, Traditional Chinese Medicine doesn't just look at your reproductive organs, and neither should you. In the Taoist worldview that gave birth to Traditional Chinese Medicine, fertility simply means the ability to bring forth something new, fresh, and exciting—to start with the nothingness of Wu Chi and create Tai Chi, Yin and Yang in perpetually changing balance, Three Treasures aligned, Five Elements in harmony. It is this exchange that is life itself, the true gift of goddesses and grandmothers.

In the spirit of Quan Yin, let us celebrate the gift of life together, whether our bodies bring forth children or our minds provide fertile ground for bright ideas. Let us recognize blessings beyond babies and miracles in myriad form. Let us not look so diligently for apples that we fail to thank the tree for producing a single perfect pear.

APPENDIX A

RECOMMENDED READING

If you want to learn more about the concepts, practices, and techniques discussed in this book, a wealth of information is available. Here are the books that we recommend in our clinic.

Acupressure
Chi Self-Massage: The Taoist Way of Rejuvenation, by Mantak Chia, Destiny Books, 2006.
Unwinding the Belly: Healing with Gentle Touch, by Allison Post and Stephen Cavaliere, North Atlantic Books, 2003.

Ba Zi
Discover Your Destiny, by Hee Yin Fan, Times Book International, 1996.

Eating and Drinking
Fertility Cycles and Nutrition, by Marilyn M. Shannon, The Couple to Couple League, 1990.
The Tao of Healthy Eating: Dietary Wisdom According to Chinese Medicine, by Bob Flaws, Blue Poppy Press, 1998.

Feng Shui
The Complete Idiot's Guide to Feng Shui, by Elizabeth Moran and Val Bikstashev, Alpha Books, 1999.

Fertility Issues
Parenting Begins Before Conception, by Carista Luminaire-Rosen, PhD, Healing Arts Press, 2000.
Taking Charge of Your Fertility, by Toni Weschler, MPH, Harper Collins, 2001.

Women's Body, Women's Wisdom, by Christiane Northrup, MD, Bantam Books, 1998.

Human Consciousness
Power vs. Force: The Hidden Determinants of Human Behavior, by David R. Hawkins, MD, PhD, Hay House, 1995.

Meditation
Awaken Healing Light of the Tao, by Mantak and Maneewan Chia, Tuttle Publishing, 1993.
Transform Stress into Vitality, by Mantak and Maneewan Chia, International Healing Tao Press, 1985.

Qi Gong and Tai Chi
Inner Structure of Tai Chi, by Mantak and Maneewan Chia, Universal Tao Publications, 1996.

Sexual Health
Cultivating Male Sexual Energy, by Mantak Chia and Maneewan Chia, Aurora Press, 1984.
Healing Love through the Tao: Cultivating Female Sexual Energy, by Mantak and Maneewan Chia, Universal Tao Publications, 1986.
The Multi-Orgasmic Couple, by Mantak Chia and Maneewan Chia, with Douglas Abrams and Rachel Carlton Abrams, MD, Harper, 2000.
The Multi-Orgasmic Man, by Mantak Chia and Douglas Abrams, Harper, 1996.
The Multi-Orgasmic Woman, by Mantak Chia and Rachel Carlton Abrams, MD, Rodale Inc., 2005.

Traditional Chinese Medicine
The Foundations of Chinese Medicine, by Giovanni Maciocia, Churchill Livingstone, 1989.

Principles of Chinese Medicine, by Angela Hicks, Thorsens, 1996.

The Web That Has No Weaver, by Ted Kaptchuk, OMD, Contemporary Books, 1975. (Includes maps showing the meridians of the body.)

APPENDIX B

MANIFESTATIONS OF THE FIVE ELEMENTS

The Five Elements are everywhere—in the world around us, in our bodies, in our spirits, in the cosmos. They govern the seasons as well as different life processes and stages of our lifetimes. We can conjure their power through the foods we eat, the emotions we cultivate, the sounds we make, and even the colors we choose to surround us. And as we do, our goal is balance, in which no single element dominates, but in which all coexist in flexible, ever-changing harmony.

The following chart explores the various qualities of the Five Elements as they manifest on Earth and in the universe.

	WOOD	FIRE	EARTH	METAL	WATER
General Aspect	Ethereal	Mind	Intellect	Corporeal	Will
Direction	East	South	Center	West	North
Stage of Development	Birth	Growth	Transformation	Harvest	Storage
Passage on Earth	Infancy	Youth	Adulthood	Old age	Death
Colors	Green	Red, pink, orange	Yellow, brown, beige	White, gold, gray, silver	Black, blue, purple
Positive Emotions	Kindness, tenderness	Joy, love, gratitude	Fairness, freedom	Courage, confidence	Gentleness, calmness
Negative Emotions	Anger, resentment, envy, jealousy	Anxiety, impatience, hatred	Worry, panic, feeling of being trapped	Depression, sadness, grief, sense of loss	Fear, insecurity, sudden fright

(continued on page 206)

	WOOD	FIRE	EARTH	METAL	WATER
Mental Aspect	Mental clarity	Intuition	Spontaneity	Emotional sensitivity	Willpower, creativity
Healing Sound	Shhh	Haaw	Vvvvvv	Ssss	Whoo
Guardian Animal	Green dragon	Red pheasant	Yellow phoenix	White tiger	Black turtle
Planet	Jupiter	Mars	Saturn	Venus	Mercury
Yin Organ	Liver	Heart	Spleen	Lungs	Kidney
Yang Organ	Gallbladder	Small intestine	Stomach	Large intestine	Bladder
Sense Organ	Eyes	Tongue	Mouth	Nose	Ear
Systems	Nervous system	Circulatory and endocrine systems	Digestive system, lymphatic system, muscles	Respiratory system	Urinary and reproductive systems
Tissues	Nail, sinew, tendon	Blood vessels	Flesh	Skin, body hair	Tooth, bone, head hair
Smell	Rancid	Burned, scorched	Fragrant	Rank, fleshy	Rotten, putrid
Taste	Sour	Bitter	Sweet	Pungent	Salty
Body Fluid	Tears	Sweat	Saliva	Phlegm	Urine
Season	Spring	Summer	Last 18 days of each season (calculated according to lunar calendar)	Spring	Winter
Weather	Wind	Heat	Dampness	Dryness	Cold
Meat	Fowl	Lamb	Beef	Venison	Pork
Grain	Wheat	Millet	Rice	Panicled millet	Beans
Human Sound	Shouting	Laughing	Singing	Weeping	Groaning
Numbers	3, 8	2, 7	5	4, 9	1, 6

APPENDIX C

COMMON PATTERNS OF DISHARMONY RELATED TO INFERTILITY

Practitioners of Traditional Chinese Medicine draw on experience and a broad body of information to diagnose and treat their patients' conditions. However, you don't need to be an expert in traditional Eastern diagnosis to apply Traditional Chinese Medicine in your own life. Simply follow the basic guidelines in chapter 2 to assess your internal weather—cooler, warmer, stagnant—by looking at your tongue and other symptoms. However, if you are interested in learning more about typical disharmony patterns related to infertility, read on.

WOMEN

The source of fertility-related disharmony in women is the Blood. To understand the exact nature of this disharmony, a practitioner of Traditional Chinese Medicine will investigate your health to determine the source of your blood disharmony: the *heart,* which powers circulation of the Blood; the *liver,* the organ that stores the blood; or the *spleen,* which governs the blood vessels that transport blood throughout the body. The following symptoms are early indicators of where a blood disharmony originates.

- **Heart disharmony:** Cold extremities, pale tongue, heart palpitations, poor circulation
- **Liver disharmony:** Mood swings, nighttime anxiety
- **Spleen disharmony:** Spotting between periods, late periods, scanty periods

As we discussed in chapter 2, Blood may be deficient, stagnant, or overheated. Symptoms described below are indicative of particular Blood disharmonies.

- **Deficient blood related to the whole body:** Pale face, lips, and tongue; dizziness or a sense of instability; overly thin body; dry skin and/or hair; scanty menstrual flow; low self-esteem; poor memory
- **Deficient blood related to the heart:** Heart palpitations, insomnia/ trouble falling asleep, anxiety, shyness, sweating, forgetfulness, feelings of vulnerability, withdrawn, afraid of speaking in public, pale face
- **Deficient blood related to the liver:** Tense, fidgety, stiff joints or tendons, spots in the field of vision, pale fingernails, absence of menstrual periods or scanty flow, irregular and/or painful periods, kind to others but unable to be compassionate toward self
- **Deficient blood related to the spleen:** Nosebleeds, unusual uterine bleeding (e.g., spotting between periods), bleeding hemorrhoids, prone to worrying or panic
- **Stagnant blood:** Stabbing pain that does not change locations, abnormal growths (e.g., cysts or fibroids), dark complexion, clotted and/or purplish menstrual blood, bruises easily, purplish tongue with red spots, inability to feel safe, excessive vigilance, suspicion, terror, or paranoia
- **Overheated blood:** Constant feeling of dryness, including dry skin; feeling thirsty no matter how much you drink; impatient or irritable; restless; plagued by nightmares; heavy periods; red skin

MEN

As we've discussed, patterns of disharmony related to fertility in men are matters of Qi—either whole-body Qi or the Qi of one of two organs most related to fertility: the lungs or the kidneys. As with women, we look for the first line of symptoms to determine if a particular organ is involved.

- **Lungs:** Very important as the source of protective Qi that supports the immune system; symptoms include respiratory, sinus, and skin problems
- **Kidneys:** Symptoms include lower back pain and erectile difficulties

Men with Qi disharmony experience Deficient Qi or its subcategory, Collapsed Qi—these are often the result of overextending ourselves energetically. However, some men experience Stagnant Qi or its subcategory, Rebellious Qi—conditions that can occur when our systems don't get enough stimulation. Symptoms of these conditions are:

- **Deficient Qi, whole body:** Consistently low energy, "couch potato" syndrome—uninterested in activity, fatigue, difficulty concentrating
- **Collapsed Qi:** When Qi is so weak it can't help maintain the body's structure—depressed, difficult to control urination, no ambition, uninspired
- **Deficient Qi, lungs:** Susceptible to colds, appears exhausted, low voice and lack of desire to talk, weak respiration, weak cough, daytime sweats, allergies, long-standing depression or grief
- **Deficient Qi, kidneys:** Edema, incontinence, frequent nighttime urination, stiff back or knees, or weak kidneys
- **Stagnant Qi:** Unlocalized pain, gas
- **Rebellious Qi:** Subcategory of stagnant Qi; when Qi moves in the wrong direction—cough, hiccups, vomiting, high blood pressure

APPENDIX D

EATING AND DRINKING WISDOM: MENU SUGGESTIONS AND RECIPES

Many couples who seek to embrace *Fertility Wisdom* find adopting its eating and drinking guidelines to be the most challenging part of the program. Yes, eating a balanced menu in harmony with the Five Elements requires most Western eaters to shift priorities, give up beloved and familiar foods (wheat, dairy, sweets, raw foods, cold drinks), and try new and unfamiliar things. But it can be done! The suggestions below will show you how.

BREAKFAST IDEAS

- 2 scrambled eggs: Scramble alone or with a little water (no milk) and cook in a little olive oil.
- 2 hard-boiled eggs: Eat with toasted spelt, oat, or soy bread if desired.
- Oatmeal: Traditional rolled oats or chewier steel-cut oats. Add dried apple slices or raisins and a small dab of honey if desired (no milk).
- 2 poached eggs and leafy greens: Sauté or steam spinach, kale, collards, or another leafy green (see recipe on page 218) to accompany the eggs.
- Meat patty and leafy greens: Sauté a patty of ground poultry (after ovulation), ground beef or lamb (if you have a cooler constitution), or ground pork (if you have a warmer constitution). Eat with greens prepared as above.
- Congee (rice soup): Prepare congee according to the recipe on page 214. For a savory breakfast, eat with chopped scallions and shredded ginger (if you have a cooler constitution), bits of meat, and cooked vegetables.

For a sweeter breakfast, add dried apple slices or raisins and a small dab of honey.

- Cottage cheese crêpes: Prepare crêpes according to the recipe on page 214. Eat with a small dab of honey.
- Breakfast burrito: Scramble eggs as above; wrap in a wheat-free tortilla.

LUNCH IDEAS

Choose from any of the breakfast options above or . . .

- Steamed white rice with meat and/or vegetables
- Rice noodles (boiled and drained) and meat and/or vegetables
- Steamed white rice with steamed or sautéed fish and/or vegetables
- Vegetable soup or vegetable miso soup if you have a warmer constitution: See recipe on page 219.
- Sautéed vegetable wrap: Sauté vegetables of your choice in olive oil with a little wheat-free tamari for seasoning. Wrap in wheat-free tortilla.

SUPPER IDEAS

Choose from any of the breakfast and lunch options above or . . .

- Sautéed peppers and portobello mushrooms, with or without meat. See recipes on page 216.
- Rice pasta with sausage: See recipe on page 216. Use chicken sausage after ovulation; otherwise use pork sausage (not too spicy). If you have a cooler constitution, don't eat too much pork, because it will cool your body. Eat with a side dish of steamed or sautéed vegetables.
- Dairy-Free Risotto with Mushrooms: See recipe on page 217. Serve with

a vegetable or add leafy greens to the risotto while it cooks.

- Beans and leafy greens: Prepare greens according to the recipe on page 218. Top with beans of your choice (e.g., white kidney beans).
- Black-bone chicken, rice or congee, and greens: Prepare the black-bone chicken according to the recipe on page 218. Prepare greens according to the recipe on page 218. Serve with steamed rice, or congee (prepared according to the recipe on page 214).

DESSERT IDEAS

Our guidelines for combining foods recommend that you skip desserts altogether (they just ferment in your stomach after a big meal, creating dampness), but if you just can't resist a little something at the end of a meal, choose your dessert carefully—for example, no refined sugar, wheat, or ice cream. (A search of the Internet will yield many wheat and sugar-free recipes, if you like to bake and can't give up desserts.)

- Fruit (in spring and summer or in a heated environment, and chosen according to your constitution). Note: Men and women of all constitutions should avoid melons of all kinds; they are very cooling.
- Low-fat cottage cheese: Enjoy with a dab of honey.
- Fertility-Friendly Fudge(less) Cake: See recipe on page 220.

SNACK IDEAS

- Low-fat cottage cheese
- Dried apple slices
- Wheat-free toast (with a little honey)
- Fruit (in spring and summer, chosen according to your constitution)
- Rice cakes
- Hummus
- Rye crackers (avoid crackers made with wheat flour)

FERTILITY-FRIENDLY RECIPES

CONGEE

1 cup long-grain white rice
1 slice ginger, optional (after ovulation)
8 cups water

Add rice (and ginger, if desired) and water to a heavy-bottomed pot (e.g., enameled cast iron). Cover the pot and bring to a gentle boil.

Immediately after the water reaches a boil, lower the temperature to its very lowest setting. Cook, covered, stirring occasionally, for 2 to 3 hours, or until the congee achieves the consistency of porridge. If the congee becomes too dry, add more water and cook a little longer.

Congee can be refrigerated, but it will congeal. To serve, add water, stir, and heat through until the congee is the desired consistency.

Remove ginger before serving.

Note: You can adjust the quantity of congee you make by following the general rule of 1 part rice to 8 parts water.

COTTAGE CHEESE CRÊPES

1 egg
⅓ cup rice flour
⅓ cup milk
1 teaspoon vanilla
Low-fat cottage cheese to fill crêpes

Whisk together the egg, rice flour, milk, and vanilla.

Melt one pat of butter in a medium skillet over low heat.

Pour in enough crêpe batter to make a 6-inch round. Increase the heat to medium.

Lift the skillet and tilt from side to side to distribute the melted butter and batter.

Flip the crêpe when the first side is done, 2 to 3 minutes.

After the second side is partially cooked, spread low-fat cottage cheese on half of the crêpe; fold over the crêpe to cover the cottage cheese.

Continue cooking 3 to 4 minutes to warm the cottage cheese.

Serve with a dab of honey.

EASY MEAT MARINADE

- 2 pieces meat (e.g., chicken breasts after ovulation only; minute steaks; pork or lamb chops), chosen according to your constitution, cleaned, and cut in strips if desired
- 1 tablespoon honey
- 1 tablespoon wheat-free tamari
- 1 tablespoon olive oil
- 1 clove garlic, crushed
- 2 scallions, chopped
- 1 slice fresh ginger (after ovulation)

In a dish, marinate the meat in the honey and tamari for ½ hour to an hour.

Heat the olive oil in a skillet. Add the garlic, scallions, and ginger (if using). Stir-fry slightly.

Add the meat, reserving the marinade, and stir-fry to brown.

Add the marinade to the skillet, reduce the heat, and simmer for about 15 minutes. Remove the ginger before serving.

SAUTÉED PEPPERS AND PORTOBELLO MUSHROOMS

2 tablespoons olive oil

1 clove garlic, chopped

4 assorted (red, yellow, and orange) bell peppers, cut into strips

2 large portobello mushrooms, cut into strips

1 tablespoon wheat-free tamari

Warm the olive oil in a skillet over medium heat. Add the garlic and sauté briefly.

Add the pepper strips; cook until softened.

Add the mushrooms and sauté.

Raise the heat slightly, add the tamari, and sauté until the liquid has been absorbed.

Serve with steamed white rice or rice noodles, with a side of meat, if desired.

RICE PASTA WITH SAUSAGE

1 package (16 ounces) rice-based pasta

3 pieces chicken sausage (after ovulation) or pork sausage (unless you have a cool constitution)

2 tablespoons olive oil

2 cloves garlic, chopped

Chopped parsley

Prepare the pasta according to package instructions.

Cut the sausage into bite-size pieces.

Warm the olive oil in a skillet over medium heat; add the garlic and sauté.

Add the sausage; brown and cook until done.

Drain the pasta and place in a large bowl. Mix in the sausage and garlic, plus a little additional olive oil, if desired.

Toss with chopped parsley.

Serve with cooked broccoli, or mix cooked broccoli into the pasta, if desired.

DAIRY-FREE RISOTTO WITH MUSHROOMS

2   tablespoons olive oil
2   cloves garlic, chopped
1   small onion, finely chopped
6   ounces sliced mushrooms
10 ounces raw Arborio or other short-grain white rice
½   cup sherry or white wine*
4   cups vegetable broth, heated
Sea salt
2   tablespoons chopped parsley

Warm the olive oil in a heavy-bottomed pan over medium heat. Add the garlic and onion and sauté until soft. Then add the mushrooms and sauté until soft.

Add the rice and stir to coat.

Pour in the wine and cook until it evaporates.

Pour in the heated broth a little at a time, stirring until the rice absorbs the liquid before adding more broth.** Add salt to taste. Stir in the chopped parsley. Allow the risotto to rest for 2 to 3 minutes before serving.

We recommend you avoid alcohol while following our Fertility Wisdom program, but because the alcohol "cooks off" in this recipe, the wine does not greatly affect the energy of the finished dish.

**To make a complete meal, stir in 2 to 3 handfuls of sliced leafy greens at this stage. Reduce the heat to low and cook until the greens are tender.*

EASY GREENS—SAUTÉED (FOR COOLER CONSTITUTIONS)

1 bunch chard, kale, spinach, or collards (not mustard greens)
2 tablespoons olive oil
2 cloves garlic, chopped
1 slice ginger—optional (after ovulation)
1 tablespoon wheat-free tamari—optional

Wash the greens. Remove woody stems. (Chop the stems and set aside if you'd like to include them in your dish.) Cut the leaves into thin strips.

Heat the olive oil in a skillet. Add the garlic and ginger (if desired) and sauté.

Add the green stems, if using, and sauté until soft but not browned.

Add the leaves and sauté until soft.

If desired, raise the heat slightly, add the tamari, and sauté until the liquid has been absorbed.

Remove the ginger before serving.

EASY GREENS—STEAMED (FOR WARMER CONSTITUTIONS)

Clean and chop the greens as above. Then, instead of sautéing, steam in a metal vegetable steamer until soft. Place the greens in a serving dish and dress with flax seed oil and a little salt before serving.

BLACK-BONE CHICKEN

1 black-bone chicken, whole*
1 bunch scallions, cut into 5 or 6 pieces (white and green parts)
5 to 6 slices gingerroot
1 tablespoon rice wine
Salt to taste

Combine all the ingredients, except salt, in an electric slow cooker or large, heavy-bottomed pot. Cover with water. Simmer on low heat for 3 to 4 hours, until chicken is tender and meat begins to come off the bone.

Serve chicken meat seasoned with salt, and a little of the cooking juice, if desired.

Black-bone chicken, sometimes sold as Silky Chicken, can be found in the frozen food section of many Asian markets. The black-bone chicken is a small bird with dark skin, a little bigger than a game hen. It is often sold with the head and feet intact.

EASY VEGETABLE SOUP

    2 tablespoons olive oil
    2 scallions, chopped, white bulb and greens separated
    1 clove garlic, chopped
    1 slice fresh ginger (after ovulation)
    1 bunch greens (such as spinach, chard, kale, or bok choy), cut into
        strips, or other vegetables as desired, cut into small pieces
        (approximately 2 cups)
    4 cups vegetable broth*
    2 tablespoons miso—optional
    Toasted white sesame seeds—optional

Heat the olive oil in a heavy-bottomed soup pot. Add the white part of the scallions, garlic, and ginger (if using). Sauté until soft but not browned.

If you're using dense vegetables (for example, broccoli or cauliflower), add them to the pot and sauté until soft.

Add the greens and sauté until soft.

Add the broth and miso (if desired) and heat through. (If using refrigerated miso paste, do not allow the soup to boil or you will destroy the active ingredients in the miso.)

While the soup is heating gently, add the green ends of the scallions. Remove the ginger, garnish with sesame seeds if desired, and serve.

If you prefer, during the post-ovulation stage of your cycle, you may substitute chicken broth.

FERTILITY-FRIENDLY FUDGE(LESS) CAKE

1 cup sifted rice flour

½ cup sifted amaranth flour

¼ cup carob powder

1 teaspoon baking soda

½ teaspoon sea salt

⅔ cup warm water*

⅓ cup vegetable oil

⅓ cup honey

1 tablespoon vinegar

1 teaspoon vanilla

Preheat the oven to 350°F. Grease one 8" or 9" square baking pan, set aside.

Sift the rice flour, amaranth flour, carob powder, baking soda, and salt together into a bowl.

Combine the water, vegetable oil, honey, vinegar, and vanilla in a small bowl and mix with a fork or whisk. Pour over the dry ingredients and mix quickly.

Pour immediately into the prepared baking pan.

Bake for 25 to 30 minutes. (Do not overbake.)

To make brownies, reduce water to ¼ cup. Spread thick batter thinly in a greased 11" × 7" or 12" × 8" pan. Bake at 350°F for 20 to 25 minutes; do not overbake.

APPENDIX E

FERTILITY-ENHANCING HERBAL FORMULAS

In our clinic, I often prescribe traditional herbal formulas to enhance fertility in my female clients. My herbal prescriptions are tailored to the specific constitution of each client I treat.

If you are working with a practitioner of Traditional Chinese Medicine, these are some of the traditional formulas he or she may prescribe. *Please do not take these or any herbal formulas without the guidance of a trained practitioner.*

Xiao Yao San (Tangkuei and Bupleurum Formula): Helps regulate menses and address PMS.

Ingredients
- Atractylodes (Alba) (Bai Zhu)
- White peony (Bai Shao)
- Poria (Fu Ling)
- Angelica root (Dang Gui)
- Bupleurum (Chai Hu)
- Ginger (brown) (Pao Jiang)
- Mint (Bo He)
- Licorice (baked) (Zhi Gan Cao)

Ba Zhen Tang (Tangkeui and Ginseng Eight Combination): Strengthens the reproductive system.

Ingredients
- Angelica root (Dang Gui)
- Ligusticum (Chuan Xiong)
- White peony (Bai Shao)

- Rehmannia (cooked) (Shu Di Huang)
- Ginseng (Ren Shen)
- Poria (Fu Ling)
- Atractylodes (Alba) (Bai Zhu)
- Ginger (fresh) (Sheng Jiang)
- Jujube (red dates) (Da Zao)
- Licorice (Gan Cao)

Bao Chan Wu You Fang (Dang Gui and Artemisia Combination): Helps secure pregnancy after conception.

Ingredients
- Angelica root (Dang Gui)
- Ligusticum root (Chuan Xiong)
- Schizonepeta bud (Jing Jie)
- Notopterygium root (Qiang Huo)
- Bitter orange fruit (Zhi Shi)
- White peony (Bai Shao)
- Dodder seeds (Tu Si Zi)
- Mugwort leaf (brown) (Ai Ye Ta)
- Astragalus root (Huang Qi)
- Fritillariae bulb (Zhe Bei Mu)
- Licorice (Can Cao)
- Ginger (fresh) (Sheng Jiang)

APPENDIX F

FERTILITY WISDOM TOOLS
AT A GLANCE

The Fertility Wisdom program offers a wide range of tools that put the power to enhance fertility in *your* hands. For a comprehensive look at these tools and how they work together, consult the chart and pages that follow.

Thank Your Body/Visualize Your Goals (page 10)

How often: Daily

Time of day: Upon rising

Constitution: All

Who: Women and men

Comments: Especially helpful when you experience physical discomfort, whether from PMS or the effects of Western fertility treatments

Affirmations (page 26)

How often: Daily

Time of day: Whenever convenient

Constitution: All

Who: Women and men

Comments: As time passes you can change your affirmations to suit your goals and state of mind. Write your affirmations down to strengthen your commitment to them and to provide a record of your fertility journey.

Connect with the Garden (page 19)

How often: When you begin the Fertility Wisdom program and daily as desired

Time of day: Upon rising

Constitution: All

Who: Women and men

Comments: Connecting with nature is a good way to ground yourself when you're stressed or distracted. Relax and bring your awareness to the physical sensations you feel while in the garden.

Pregnancy Readiness Survey and Partner Exercises (page 51)

How often: When you begin the Fertility Wisdom program

Time of day: Whenever you and your partner can dedicate undivided attention to the task

Constitution: All

Who: Women and men

Comments: Choose a time when you and your partner are not stressed, in an emotionally charged situation, or distracted (for example, not while driving). Write down your answers so you can revisit them as your fertility journey unfolds.

Read Your Tongue/Check Your Constitution (page 43)

How often: Daily

Time of day: Upon rising—before drinking, eating, or brushing teeth—and as necessary throughout the day

Constitution: All

Who: Women and men

Comments: Consulting your tongue's "weather report" should be a regular part of your day. Do it first thing in the morning, and especially after any changes in environment, emotional state, or eating and drinking patterns. Pay attention to how your body feels—for example, do you have sensations of heat or cold? is your digestion upset?—and check your tongue for a constitutional update when you notice changes. If you cannot identify your constitution by looking at your tongue and assessing other physical indicators, consult a practitioner of Traditional Chinese Medicine for assistance or follow guidelines for a neutral/balanced constitution.

Exercise

How often: Regularly—customized to your constitution and where you are in your menstrual cycle/pregnancy

Time of day: Pay attention to how your body responds to exercise and time your activities accordingly. For example, if exercise relaxes you, exercise later in the day; if it energizes you, choose a morning time.

Constitution: All

Who: Women and men

Comments: If possible, work with a practitioner of Traditional Chinese Medicine or a personal trainer to develop a personalized exercise regimen that supports conception and pregnancy. Avoid vigorous physical exercise after ovulation and during the first trimester of pregnancy. Warmer constitutions should be take care to avoid over-exercising.

Rest/Sleep

How often: Regularly, according to body's needs

Time of day: Nighttime, and daytime (e.g., naps, restful meditation) as necessary to maintain a balanced constitution

Constitution: All

Who: Women and men

Comments: To determine how much rest or sleep you need, pay close attention to the messages your mind and body send you. If you are stressed, overheated, overworked, or over-exercised, make getting more rest and restful sleep a top priority.

Eating and Drinking (page 77)

How often: Regularly

Time of day: Meal and snack times to suit your body's needs

Constitution: All, with consumption customized to your constitution.

Who: Women and men

Comments: After reading your tongue and noting other physical signs to determine if your body is warmer, cooler, or experiencing stagnation, consult the food and beverage charts in chapter 000 to customize a meal plan to your constitution. Note that your constitutional "weather" may change day to day, or even throughout the day, so adjust your intake of food and beverage accordingly. Most important—learn to drink and eat *before* you become thirsty or hungry; don't wait until you're dehydrated or ravenous.

Ama's Poached Eggs (page 71)

How often: Once monthly, when all menstrual bleeding has ceased, while you are preparing your body for pregnancy

Time of day: On an empty stomach

Constitution: Not for warmer constitutions or constitutions with stagnation

Who: Women

Comments: Enjoy Ama's Poached Eggs for breakfast after all menstrual bleeding has ceased. Discontinue during months when you are trying to become pregnant to avoid over-warming your body.

Eat Organic Poultry (page 74)

> **How often:** After ovulation if you think you're pregnant and throughout pregnancy—in moderation. Unless you are preparing your body for pregnancy and eating Ama's Poached Eggs after menstruation, avoid poultry during the first half of your cycle.
>
> **Time of day:** As desired
>
> **Constitution:** If your body shows signs of heat or stagnation be cautious—don't overdo; poultry's constricting energy may intensify a warmer or stagnant constitution.
>
> **Who:** Women
>
> **Comments:** As with all foods, pay attention to how your body reacts when you eat poultry. If you notice signs of overheating or stagnation, cut back. (See also notes on consumption of Black Chicken.)

Eat "Black Chicken" (page 218)

> **How often:** In moderation
>
> **Time of day:** As desired
>
> **Constitution:** All—particularly good for constitutions that need nourishment (e.g., low sperm count/motility in men, women with thin uterine lining)
>
> **Who:** Women and men
>
> **Comments:** Black chicken, available in the frozen food section of many Asian grocery stores, has different energetic properties from regular poultry, which has a constricting energy. Black chicken's water-element energy makes it particularly beneficial to the reproductive systems of both women and men.

Vitamin/Mineral Supplements (page 96)

> **How often:** Daily
>
> **Time of day:** With meals or as instructed by nutritionist/

physician/practitioner of Traditional Chinese Medicine

Constitution: All

Who: Women and men

Comments: See guidelines in chapter 000 regarding supplements and/or consult with a nutritionist or practitioner of Traditional Chinese Medicine to customize a regimen to your needs. (At the very least, take the prenatal vitamins recommended by your Western doctor.)

Feel Qi Ball/Bring Qi to Hands (page 34)

How often: Daily

Time of day: Upon rising

Constitution: All

Who: Women and men

Comments: In addition to being a good way to start the day, this exercise is a helpful way to get in touch with your body when you're feeling ungrounded or emotional. It's also a warm-up exercise before during acupressure.

Uterus Lift (page 110)

How often: At least twice a day; women should discontinue after ovulation if there's the possibility of pregnancy and/or during the first trimester of pregnancy.

Time of day: Upon rising or before falling asleep, after Groin Pulse Acupressure; and/or after urinating. (If you do the Uterus Lift while lying down be sure your knees are higher than your hips.)

Constitution: All

Who: Women (and men—see instructions)

Comments: This is an excellent exercise for women to resume after the birth of a baby and beyond for general reproductive health. And men can gain benefits from regularly performing a "lift" tailored to their anatomy.

Open Wind Gates (page 106)

How often: Daily

Time of day: Any time of day but perhaps most convenient upon rising or before falling asleep, when you're already lying down, after Groin Pulse Acupressure and Wind Gates, with knees higher than hips.

Constitution: All

Who: Women and men

Comments: Discontinue all Wind Gate points below the navel after ovulation when there's the possibility of pregnancy and during the first trimester of pregnancy.

Groin Pulse Acupressure (page 112)

How often: 2 times each day

Time of day: Upon rising and before falling asleep, before performing the Uterus Lift, Wind Gates, or other exercises, with knees flat.

Constitution: All

Who: Women and men

Comments: If you feel fatigue in your back or legs, do Groin Pulse Acupressure more frequently.

Inner Smile Meditation (page 117)

How often: Daily

Time of day: Morning or evening

Constitution: All

Who: Women and men

Comments: May be performed while sitting, lying down, or standing. Pay attention to how your body reacts to the Inner Smile. If this meditation relaxes you, do it in the evening; if it energizes you, do it in the morning. Follow with Microcosmic Orbit Meditation.

Microcosmic Orbit Meditation (page 122)

How often: Daily

Time of day: Following Inner Smile Meditation

Constitution: All

Who: Women and men

Comments: May be performed while sitting, lying down, or standing. Follows Inner Smile Meditation.

Six Healing Sounds (page 123)

How often: At least once a day, more as needed

Time of day: Morning, evening, or whenever needed

Constitution: All—especially warmer constitutions

Who: Women and men

Comments: The Six Healing Sounds can be performed sitting, lying down—even while walking around (subvocally, without the postures). This exercise is especially helpful when you feel stressed, overextended, or overheated.

Qi Gong warm up (page 133)

How often: Daily or 3 times per week

Time of day: Upon rising is best, but if these exercises relax rather than energize you, perform them in the evening.

Constitution: All

Who: Women and men

Comments: The Qi Gong Warmup exercises may be

performed as a sequence unto themselves or as part of a larger sequence that includes Intensive Qi Gong and Cool Down.

Intensive Qi Gong (page 147)

How often: Daily or three times per week

Time of day: Morning or evening

Constitution: All

Who: Women (Ovarian Breathing), Women and Men (Tapping Perineum Power)

Comments: Perform after Qi Gong Warmup exercises and before Qi Gong Cool down. Do not perform after ovulation or if you are pregnant. If you have high blood pressure or if your blood pressure rises with exercise, do not do the Tapping Perineum Power exercise; instead simply meditate for a moment, bringing your awareness to the perineum. If your menstrual cycle tends to be longer than 28 days or if bleeding during your period is very light (or if you do not menstruate at all), do not do Ovarian Breathing.

Qi Gong Cool-down (page 152)

How often: Daily or three times per week to conclude the full Qi Gong sequence (including Warmup and Intensive Qi Gong)

Time of day: Morning or evening

Constitution: All

Who: Women and men

Comments: You can do this exercise any time you feel overstimulated or to relax/cool down after other types of exercise, like walking)

Sun Bathing (page 153)

How often: No more than 3 times per week

Time of day: See instructions

Constitution: Cooler constitutions only. (In particular, men with warmer constitutions should not do this exercise)

Who: Women and men

Comments: It's very important that you sunbathe for no more than 15 minutes at a time to avoid overheating and compromising your reproductive system.

Moxibustion (page 156)

How often: Daily

Time of day: When convenient

Constitution: If you have a warmer constitution consult a practitioner of Traditional Chinese Medicine before using moxa

Who: Women

Comments: Follow instructions carefully to determine appropriate points for moxibustion before and after ovulation and to avoid burning yourself.

Ginger Moxa for Scars (page 161)

How often: Daily

Time of day: When convenient

Constitution: For cooler constitutions only

Who: Women

Comments: Discontinue ginger moxa if you feel overheated, after ovulation, and during pregnancy.

Feng Shui Adjustments (page 163)

How often: Before beginning the Fertility Wisdom program, with periodic checks to reduce clutter and keep your environment conducive to conception and pregnancy

Time of day: When convenient

Constitution: All

Who: Women and men

Comments: If you can only make Feng Shui adjustments in
one location, make it your bedroom.

Post-Ovulation/First Trimester "Don'ts"

From the first day of ovulation through the first day of menstruation—and
during the first trimester of pregnancy—avoid:

Travel via air or by car on bumpy roads

Vigorous exercise

Exercise that activates the PC muscle (e.g., Kegel exercises,
Uterine Lift, stair and hill climbing)

Vigorous sexual activity

Hot or cold baths (okay if body temperature and no more than
15 minutes)

Hot or cold showers

Swimming

Intense emotional experiences

Scented products

Ginger juice/dried ginger

Wind Gates below the navel

Ginger moxa (on scars)

Special note: Be sure to use different points for moxibustion before and
after ovulation. See moxibustion guidelines on page 158 for more information.

INDEX

Boldface page references indicate illustrations.
Underscored references indicate boxed text.